Taking Control

Living with the Mitral Valve Prolapse Syndrome

Kristine A. Bludau Scordo, Ph.D., R.N., C.N.P., A.C.N.P.

Professor and Director, Acute Care Nurse Practitioner Program,
Wright State University, Dayton, Ohio

Cardiology Acute Care Nurse Practitioner,
Schuster Associates Cardiology, Dayton, Ohio

Former Clinical Director,
The Mitral Valve Prolapse Program of Cincinnati,
Cincinnati, Ohio

THIRD EDITION
REVISED AND UPDATED

KARDINAL PUBLISHING
CINCINNATI, OHIO
2007

Taking Control: Living with the Mitral Valve Prolapse Syndrome, 3rd edition

Publishing History
First edition: 1991 Copyright © Camden House, Inc.
Second edition: 1996 Copyright © K.A. Bludau Scordo.

Graphic images © New Vision Technologies Inc.

Published by Kardinal Publishing
Designed and produced by GYAT
Edited by Justine Cullinan

Printed in the United States of America by Perfection Printing, Cincinnati, OH
ISBN 978-1-4243-1576-5

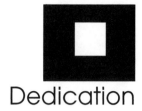

Dedication

To those with mitral valve prolapse.

May it do you much good
— ABRAHAM KAPLAN, 1964

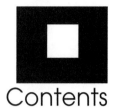

Contents

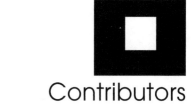

Contributors
and Consultants

1st, 2nd & 3rd Editions

Kristine A. Bludau Scordo Ph.D., R.N., C.N.P., A.C.N.P.
Professor and Director of the Acute Care Nurse Practitioner Program, Wright State University, Dayton, Ohio; former Clinical Director, The Mitral Valve Prolapse Program of Cincinnati; Cardiology Acute Care Nurse Practitioner, Schuster Cardiology, Dayton, Ohio

Linda Hussey, M.S.N., R.N., C.S., L.P.C.C.
Clinical Nurse Specialist; Psychiatric nursing; private practice, Cincinnati, Ohio

1st & 2nd Editions

LeOna Kriesel Cox, B.S. Education
Educator and author; former teacher, Economics Department, Allegheny College, Meadville, Pennsylvania; author of educational texts and filmstrip scripts

1st Edition

Fuheid S. Daoud, M.D.
Cardiologist; Medical Director, The Cardiology Center of Cincinnati; The Mitral Valve Prolapse Program of Cincinnati, The Health Promotion and Rehabilitation Center, Cincinnati, Ohio

Linda Harte Hoffsis, M.A.
Exercise Physiologist and Registered Dietician; Coordinator of the Cardiac Rehabilitation Program, Health Promotion and Rehabilitation Center, Cincinnati, Ohio; Staff Exercise Physiologist, MVP Program of Cincinnati

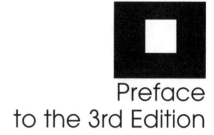

Preface
to the 3rd Edition

This edition brings new information compiled from data obtained from recent research on the mitral valve prolapse syndrome (MVPS). The first study, entitled "Factors Associated with Participation in a Mitral Valve Prolapse Support Group," was funded by Wright State University (WSU) and involved MVP support group participants. This study explored the characteristics of individuals who are most likely to benefit from and participate in a support group, and determined the important aspects of a support group. The second study, entitled "Mitral Valve Prolapse Syndrome: Health Concerns, Role Function and Health Service Use," was funded by Grant R15 NR07997-01 from the Department of Health and Human Services (DHHS), National Institutes of Heath (NIH), National Institute of Nursing Research (NINR). The purpose of this study was to develop a profile of health concerns, symptoms, and treatments, and to examine the relationships of symptoms to role status and use of health-care services for patients diagnosed with mitral valve prolapse syndrome (MVPS). Information obtained from participants helped to answer questions such as: What are the health concerns, symptoms, and treatments reported by patients with MVPS? Are health concerns related to age, time since diagnosis, symptoms, anxiety, social support, diet (magnesium, sodium, water and caffeine), and treatment (beta- and calcium-channel blockers; anxiolytics; meditation/relaxation therapy; exercise; activity limitation)? Data from more than a thousand individuals diagnosed with MVPS, from every state in the U.S. and from several foreign countries, provided further insight into MVPS. These studies, along with an updated review of the literature on topics related to MVPS, are incorporated into various chapters in this third edition. For those people who wish further information, references are listed at the end of each chapter.

Once again, this updated edition would not be possible without the help of several individuals. I am grateful to the many WSU graduate nursing students, faculty, and staff who assisted with either the research studies or by reviewing the literature for specific chapters. They are DeAnne Colvard French, Ph.D. and Harry Khamis, Ph.D., statistical consultants; Joyce Marrs, M.S., R.N., C.N.P., Heather Caskey, M.S., R.N., C.N.P., and Charlene Callahan, M.S., R.N. for help with the NIH, NINR study; Cindy White, M.S., R.N., C.N.P. for advice for Chapter 4; Michelle Weaver, M.S., R.N., C.N.P., for advice for Chapter 10; Karen Beth Clark, M.S., R.N., C.N.P. and José W. Almeyda, B.S.N., R.N., for advice for Chapter 11. I am grateful to Linda Hussey, M.S., R.N. for her thoughtful review and critique of Chapter 7. I am also indebted to Ximena Chrisagis, M.S. (LIS), M.A., AHIP, Health Sciences Librarian at WSU, for being a tremendous resource in securing articles for this edition. A special thanks also goes to Nalda Blair, administrative secretary for the Acute Care Nurse Practitioner program at WSU for her incredible assistance—she truly is a "jack of all trades."

I am deeply grateful my sister Stephanie J. Bludau Tor for guiding this book through the press and to her colleague Justine Cullinan for her editing and proofreading.

This book is dedicated to my best investment, my daughter, Lisa Jacobsen, and to her husband Eric and my two wonderful grandsons, Noah and Liam. I cherish their love and support.

— *Kristine Scordo*

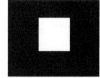

Foreword to the First Edition

Taking Control: Living with the MVPS is intended to help individuals to cope with the myriad of symptoms associated with MVPS. Those of us in the medical field who frequently diagnose people with this syndrome recognize the enormous and time-consuming difficulty in dealing with the disproportionate perception of these individuals of the serious nature of their symptoms. They are understandably frightened by chest pain, alarmed by palpitations, dizziness, and light-headedness, and frustrated by unexplained fatigue, moodiness, and anxiety attacks.

I am afraid that we as physicians have failed to adequately handle the needs of the large number of people with this syndrome, mainly because of the inordinate amount of time it takes to do so. Explaining the common denominator in this syndrome, namely the anatomically variant structure of the valve and support structures, is an easy task. Explaining the varied and multiple associated symptoms, however, is a difficult one. Reassuring these individuals that the chest pain is not necessarily a prelude to a fatal heart attack, that the palpitations are not a signal of a life-threatening arrhythmia, and that the fatigue, tiredness, and headache are not symptoms of underlying serious illness requires a separate and distinct discussion.

Kris Scordo has succeeded in meeting this challenge in *Taking Control*. In addition to her own enormous contribution based on experience gained over several years of clinical experience and research for her doctoral dissertation, she was able to enlist the talent and expertise of others who for years also patiently and tirelessly worked with individuals with this syndrome. She and her colleagues have addressed various aspects of this syndrome, making this book the most comprehensive to date. Individuals with this syndrome should, after reading this book, be able to put the syndrome in proper perspective. I look forward to making it available to every person diagnosed with this syndrome.

—Fuheid S. Daoud, M.D.

1

Understanding the Mitral Valve Prolapse Syndrome

"I'm only 25 years old. How could I be having a heart attack?"
"I was given no explanation other than 'don't worry'."
"We would race to the hospital only to be sent home."
"I was beginning to believe I was crazy—it was all in my head."
"I feel like a second-class citizen. How come no one is taking this seriously?"

The story is all too familiar. First, you search for a diagnosis. After several visits with a physician and multiple tests, you're finally given a reason for the symptoms, and then told—don't worry. Now the questions begin. "What do I have? Mitral valve what? What does that mean? Will it get worse? Does my valve have to be replaced? Am I having a heart attack because I have chest pain? Will this affect my pregnancy? Is this common? How can I feel better?"

More than likely, you had similar thoughts and questions when you were first diagnosed with mitral valve prolapse (MVP). Perhaps you still have a number of questions. Let me begin by telling you, you are not alone. You are among millions of people with MVP—or MVPers.

Mitral valve prolapse (MVP) was once believed to be a very common clinical entity with reported prevalences from 2% to 22%. Initial data from the Framingham Heart Study, a prospective epidemiological investigation begun in 1948, estimated a prevalence of 7.6% in women and 2.5% in men. Recent studies, however, indicate that the prevalence of MVP in the United States is estimated at 2.4% with no gender differences. This is based on recent analysis of data from the offspring cohort of the Framingham Heart Study. The much higher and wider range of prevalences in initial studies reflects variations in the methods used to diagnosis MVP [auscultation and/or echocardiographic (heart ultrasound) criteria] and the composition of the study population (age, race, gender). Recent studies use very specific echocardiographic criteria, which may partly explain the lower prevalence rates. How many people with symptomatic mitral valve prolapse syndrome remain unknown?

Mitral valve prolapse is believed to be inherited in an autosomal dominant mode. In this mode of inheritance, one parent has the disease and transmits the gene to one or more offspring. Interestingly, in a study of 1,752 newborns, mitral valve prolapse was not seen on echocardiograms, nor were there any heart sounds indicative of MVP. This study suggests that MVP is an acquired disease with no significant clinical expression at birth. Thus, the development of MVP may depend on age or be influenced by environmental factors. In fact, sex- and age-dependent penetrance, or the extent to which a genetically determined condition is expressed in an individual, has been noted. MVP was more prevalent in young adult females than in children, and it increased with age. In the more recent Framingham Heart Study, however, there was a fairly even distribution (2–3%) of MVP among persons in each decade of age from 30 to 80 years. Furthermore, striking differences in valvular abnormalities can be seen in family members who inherit the MVP gene. For instance, a sister might have mild prolapse of the mitral valve, whereas her brother has severe prolapse.

Although people with MVP come in all shapes and sizes, there are physical features commonly associated with MVP. These include: pectus excavatum (depression of the breast bone), scoliosis (curvature of the spine), abnormally straight thoracic spine (straight back), arm span greater than height, unusual joint flexibility and low body weight.

Mitral valve prolapse has been around for a long time. In fact, symptoms similar to MVP syndrome have been traced back to the 1600s. MVP has been known by a variety of names including irritable heart, soldier's heart, the effort syndrome, Barlow's syndrome, and DaCosta's syndrome. British solders during the mid-1800s noted symptoms of fatigue, palpitations, shortness of breath, and chest pain, and were unable to perform demanding physical tasks. This was a major cause of medical disability. Similar findings were noted during the Civil War, World War I, and World War II.

William Osler, an eminent physician, noted the similarity between symptoms associated with irritable heart mentioned by others and those occurring in the general population, particularly in women. Some physicians believed the problem was not the heart, but one of a psychiatric nature. As technology advanced, so did the understanding of mitral valve prolapse. The 1980s saw the development of the classification of mitral valve prolapse into anatomic MVP and the MVP syndrome.

Normal Heart Function

The heart is a hollow muscular organ whose function is to pump blood. The right side of the heart pumps blood to the lungs and the left side pumps blood to the rest of the body. The right and left sides of the heart each have an upper chamber (atrium), which collects blood and pumps it into a lower chamber (ventricle), which pumps blood out. Four heart valves allow blood to flow in one direction. Each valve consists of leaflets or flaps that open and close like one-way swinging doors. The mitral valve has two cusps, while the other values—tricuspid, aortic, and pulmonary—have three. The mitral and tricuspid valves have tethers that consist of papillary muscles and supporting cords that prevent the valves from swinging backward into the atria. The competence of the mitral valve apparatus is dependent on the structural and functional integrity of the leaflets, annulus, chordae tendineae, papillary muscles and wall of the heart muscle (myocardium).

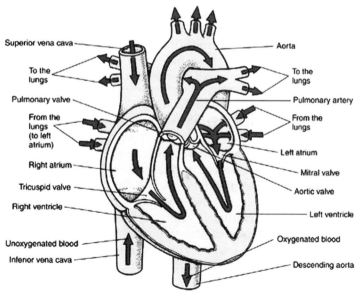

Anatomic Mitral Valve Prolapse

Anatomic mitral valve prolapse is an abnormality of the mitral valve apparatus (valve leaflets and support chords). These structures allow the leaflet(s) to prolapse—buckle back into the left atrium during the heart's contraction, or ventricular systole. The most common and clinically important structural change is mitral valve leaflet thickening and redundancy, known as myxomatous degeneration. In myxomatous degeneration, the structural proteins abnormally form and cause thickening, enlargement and redundancy of the leaflets and supporting chords (chordae tendineae). When the ventricle contracts, the redundant leaflet(s) prolapses into the left atrium, and sometimes may allow leakage or backflow of blood through the valve opening (mitral regurgitation) into the left atrium. This backflow of blood can be mild, moderate, or severe.

Anatomic MVP can be further defined as classic or nonclassic prolapse. Classic prolapse is prolapse with at least 5 mm (~0.20″) thickening of the valve leaflets, whereas nonclassic prolapse has lesser degrees of leaflet thickening. Studies implicate leaflet thickening as an indicator of prognosis; individuals with classic MVP appear to have a higher risk for complications than do those with leaflets less than 2 mm in thickness.

Several mechanisms can produce MVP. When the cause of the prolapse cannot be identified, it is described as *primary* mitral valve prolapse. When MVP is a consequence of other conditions, it is known as *secondary* mitral valve prolapse. One example of secondary mitral valve prolapse is prolapse caused by endocarditis—a bacterial infection of the valve. Please note that this book will discuss *primary* mitral valve prolapse.

Mitral Valve Prolapse Syndrome

Primary anatomic mitral valve prolapse is frequently associated with a constellation of symptoms. Individuals with one or more of these symptoms are referred to as having the mitral valve prolapse *syndrome*—MVPS. The term MVP syndrome refers to the occurrence of, or coexistence of, symptoms unexplainable on the basis of the valvular abnormality. *Thus, the symptoms associated with MVPS are not due to the valve itself.* They are believed to be based on various physiological changes. These are discussed later.

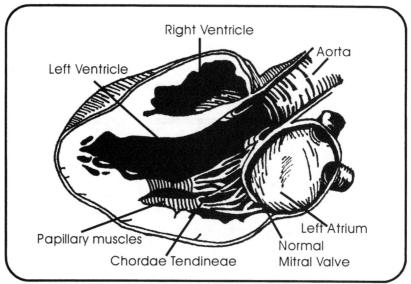

NORMAL MITRAL VALVE

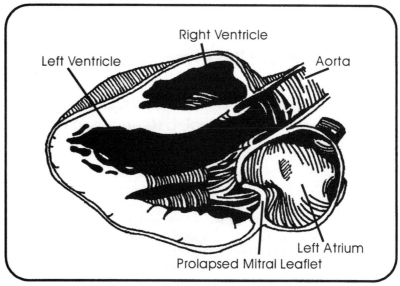

PROLAPSE OF THE MITRAL VALVE

Common symptoms are listed in Table 1-1. This table is compiled from data from 837 individuals diagnosed with MVPS. Symptoms are listed according to their frequency.

TABLE 1-1. MITRAL VALVE PROLAPSE SYNDROME:
COMMON SYMPTOMS (N = 837)

	N	%
Palpitations	708	87
Anxiety	634	79
Skipped beats	626	75
Fatigue	619	74
Lightheadedness	584	70
Chest pain	554	66
Panic attacks	494	59
Shortness of breath	486	58
Extra beats	473	56
Dizziness	433	52
Mood swings	397	47
Headaches	395	48
Tachycardia	337	40
Other	204	24
Passing out	87	10

Characteristics of the Symptoms

Palpitations, Skipped Beats, Extra Heart Beats, Forceful Heart Beat, Pounding Heart, Heart Flutter, Tachycardia

People describe palpitations—extra beats—as a pounding sensation in their chest. Others say they feel a flip-flop or fluttering. Arrhythmias—disturbances in the heart rhythm—such as atrial extra beats (PACs) or premature ventricular extrasystoles (PVCs) can cause palpitations. While some people feel each beat, others do not notice them. Often, after extra beats, people have a sensation that their heart stopped for a few seconds.

Skipped or extra beats are very common among MVPers *and* the general public. Sometimes they occur following the use of caffeine, alcohol, tobacco, or certain medications. Other times,

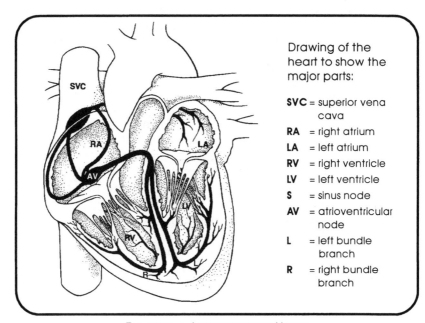

Drawing of the heart to show the major parts:

SVC = superior vena cava

RA = right atrium

LA = left atrium

RV = right ventricle

LV = left ventricle

S = sinus node

AV = atrioventricular node

L = left bundle branch

R = right bundle branch

ELECTRICAL ACTIVITY OF THE HEART

emotional stress may cause extra beats. Sometimes they happen for no apparent reason. In any case, these beats are relatively common, and should not be a cause for alarm. An explanation of the heart's electrical system may help to understand extra beats.

Each heartbeat normally starts in the right atrium. Here, a specialized group of cells called the sinus node—natural pacemaker—sets the pace for the heart's rhythm. From the sinus node, the electrical impulse spreads across the atria—the top

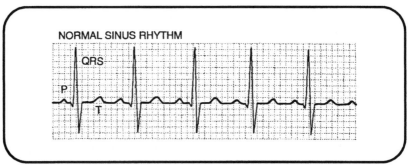

NORMAL SINUS RHYTHM

QRS

P

T

EKG TRACING

part of the heart. This activity registers on the electrocardiogram (EKG) in the form of a blip, called the P wave. As the electrical impulse travels down the specialized conduction system to the ventricles, a QRS complex is generated.

As the electrical signal travels through the heart, the heart contracts. First, the atria—top chambers— contract, pumping blood into the ventricles. A fraction of a second later, the ventricles—bottom chambers—contract, sending blood throughout the body. After each contraction, the heart relaxes for a brief moment. This relaxation produces the T wave on the EKG.

The heart normally contracts between 60 and 100 times per minute. Each contraction equals one heartbeat. This series of events occurs over 100,000 times a day. Alterations in the normal electrical sequence result in arrhythmias—disturbances in the heart rhythm.

There are many types of arrhythmias. Arrhythmias are identified by *where* they occur in the heart, and by *what happens* to the heart's rhythm when they occur. Arrhythmias sometimes originate in the atria or ventricles. They sometimes occur as a

TESTS FOR DETECTING ARRHYTHMIAS

- *Resting Electrocardiogram*: While the patient is at rest, disks or electrodes are placed on the chest, arms, and legs and a recording is made.

- *Graded Exercise Stress Test*: Exercise on a treadmill machine or bicycle while connected to the EKG machine.

- *24-hour Holter Monitor*: Ambulatory monitor that records the EKG over a period of 24 hours.

- *Trans-telephone or Event Monitor*: A monitoring device worn from several days to several weeks. When the arrhythmia is felt, it is transmitted over the phone and the EKG recorded, or stored in the monitor's memory and transmitted at a later time.

- *Electrophysiologic Study*: An invasive test that involves cardiac catheterization. Thin, flexible tubes—catheters—are placed in an arm or leg vein and advanced to the heart. This allows for special recordings to be made.

single beat or as repeated periods of very fast heartbeats. When a beat occurs early in the atria, it is known as a premature atrial beat or contraction. An atrial tachycardia occurs when a series of early atrial beats increase the heart rate. In paroxysmal tachycardia, repeated periods of very fast heartbeats begin and end suddenly.

Arrhythmias can be detected by listening to the heart with a stethoscope. An arrhythmia may not be present, however, at the time of the examination. Therefore, other tests are needed to detect the arrhythmia. The type of test depends on how often the arrhythmia occurs, and in what setting. For example, if activity brings on the arrhythmia, a graded exercise stress test is indicated. Otherwise, if the arrhythmia occurs infrequently, an event monitor would be appropriate.

Premature ventricular contractions are common in MVPers. PVCs originate from an electrical signal in the ventricles, and occur prematurely in the cardiac cycle. Depending upon the prematurity of the PVC, it may not allow the heart enough time to fill with blood. This causes an ineffective contraction. Therefore, the heart doesn't pump its full requirement of blood. After the premature ventricular beat, sometimes a sensation occurs that the heart stopped. To understand this sensation, think of the heart as a large rubber band. The greater you stretch the rubber band, the harder it springs back. When a beat is premature and the heart doesn't have adequate time to fill with blood, the rubber band—heart muscle—stretches a little and doesn't bounce back as much. The heart, therefore, doesn't do the same amount of work, or pump the same amount of blood. If you take your pulse, you don't feel the premature beat.

Next, the heart pauses—a compensatory pause—to compensate for the prematurity of PVC. This pause causes the sensation that the heart has stopped. It allows the heart more time to fill with blood. Therefore, the rubber band stretches farther, and the heart's contraction becomes more forceful—the "flip-flop" feeling. It is the beat *after* the extra beat that most people feel.

When people describe palpitations, or a forceful heart beat, arrhythmias may not be noted. What may be felt is sinus tachycardia—a speeding up of the natural heart beat. Every day, almost everyone has periods when their rate exceeds 100 beats per minute. Exercise, anxiety, and secret rendezvous with your lover naturally increase your heart rate. Too, when you are out of shape—deconditioned—and running up a flight of stairs, your heart rapidly pounds.

TYPES OF ARRHYTHMIAS

- *Sinus tachycardia*: A speeding up of the natural pacemaker of the heart to rates over 100 beats per minute.

- *Sinus bradycardia*: A slowing down of the natural pacemaker of the heart to rates less than 60 beats per minute.

- *Premature atrial contraction*: A beat that occurs early in the atria and causes the heart to beat prematurely.

- *Paroxysmal supraventricular tachycardia* (PSVT): A series of repeated beats that originate above the ventricles and speed up the heart rate. Usually PSVT begins and ends suddenly.

- *Atrial fibrillation*: Electrical signals in the atria fire multiple electrical impulses. A fraction of these impulses make their way down to the ventricles in an irregular fashion. This makes the pulse rate very irregular.

- *Premature ventricular contraction* (PVC): An electrical signal from the ventricles that causes the heart to beat before the next regular heartbeat.

- *Ventricular tachycardia*: Three or more premature ventricular contractions that occur together.

- *Ventricular fibrillation*: Electrical signals are fired from the ventricles in a very fast and chaotic manner. This causes the heart to lose its ability to pump blood.

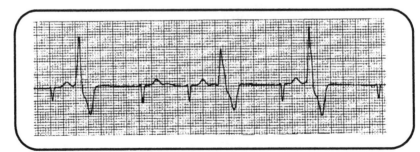

PREMATURE VENTRICULAR CONTRACTIONS

There is often a discordance between the EKG and the person's *sensations* of extra beats or *sensations* of a pounding heart. During 24-hour Holter monitor recordings, MVPers record palpitations in the diary, and believe they have an arrhythmia. When the EKG tracings are reviewed, only sinus tachycardia is noted.

Anxiety and/or Panic Attacks

Although the relationship is not clear, many MVPers suffer from anxiety or panic attacks. The symptoms described are more consistent with panic disorder, the anxiety disorder studied most often in MVP patients. People have recurrent, spontaneous anxiety attacks that consist of various combinations of symptoms similar to some MVPS symptoms. These symptoms include: fatigue, fainting, dizziness, chest pain, lightheadedness, rapid heartbeat, heart palpitations, and shortness of breath.

The degree and mechanism of association between MVPS and anxiety disorders remains unclear. While some believe the symptoms cause anxiety attacks, others believe extraneous factors trigger attacks. They may occur anywhere, at anytime, even in the middle of the night. Whenever anxiety attacks do occur, they are frightening.

Fatigue

Fatigue is usually present to some degree. It may be episodic and severe, or relatively constant. Usually fatigue begets more fatigue—the less you do, the less you feel like doing. The cause of the fatigue may relate to blood volume changes noted with exercise, to a high resting heart rate, or to other physiological factors to be discussed shortly.

Lightheadedness, Dizziness

Lightheadedness, dizziness, or both can occur when first standing up. This feeling is usually associated with a sensation of a forceful heart beat or palpitations. More specifically, postural orthostatic tachycardia syndrome (POTS) is present when orthostatic intolerance (i.e., symptoms on standing that are relieved by recumbency) occur in the presence of a demonstrable exaggerated, persistent postural sinus tachycardia (greater than 30 bpm from baseline or greater than 120 bpm) that occurs within 2–5 minutes of assuming an upright posture. These symptoms may be related to a decreased intravascular volume and autonomic dysfunction.

Chest Pain

The chest pain associated with MVP presents itself in many ways. The pain may be brief in duration or persist for hours. People describe the pain as sharp, heavy, shooting, sticking, or as pressure. At times it can be incapacitating, occurring repeatedly. Often the chest pain is atypical of angina—pain caused by narrowing or constriction in the coronary arteries. Sometimes, however, the pain mimics angina.

Many MVPers believe chest pains signal a heart attack. MVPS is not known to cause a heart attack. In general, severe narrowing and blockage of a coronary artery that supplies an area of heart muscle with blood causes a heart attack. This may lead to permanent damage of a portion of the heart muscle. MVPS neither narrows nor blocks coronary arteries, nor causes permanent damage to the heart muscle.

You ask, "How can I be sure the chest pain is not from coronary artery disease?" The answer to this relates to your original diagnosis. To first determine whether heart disease is present, your physician considers your cardiovascular risk factors such as age, sex, family history, blood lipid profile, and smoking history, as well as your symptoms and results of diagnostic testing. Periodically, he or she follows up with testing such as an exercise stress test to reassure you that the chest pain is not caused by coronary artery disease.

Shortness of Breath

This is usually described as the inability to take in a deep breath. It may occur at rest or with activity. The shortness of breath has not been found to be related to heart or lung abnormalities.

Mood Swings

Mood swings, or an emotional state that alternates between periods of euphoria and depression, are described by many MVPers of all ages. One minute you're feeling on top of the world, and the next you're ready to "go ballistic." Mood swings have a certain knack for making you feel completely lost. In fact, many people believe that their behavior is totally incomprehensible and beyond their control. This may not be the case as you will learn in Chapter 7, *Anxiety, Panic Attacks, and MVPs*.

Causes of mood swings are likely multifactorial. They may be related to or associated with sleep disturbances, premenstrual syndrome (PMS), perimenopause, menopause, post-partum depression, anxiety or depressive disorders, certain drugs or alcohol, or merely may represent an improper use of the term. Frequent and rapidly shifting moods, however, may be a sign of a personality disorder that requires further diagnosis and treatment. Although detailed discussion of personality disorders is beyond the scope of this book, according to the American Psychiatric Association (APA), the essential feature of borderline personality disorder is a pervasive pattern of instability of interpersonal relationships, affects, and self-image, as well as marked impulsivity. These characteristics begin by early adulthood and are present in a variety of contexts. (Further information is available at the APA website: www.psych.org.Society).

Headaches

Headaches sometimes occur in the form of migraines and are accompanied by nausea and blurred vision. Some people describe their headaches as nagging or dull.

Other Symptoms

MVPers report other symptoms. Common ones include:
- Chronically cold hands and feet
- Gastrointestinal (stomach) disturbances
- Problems with memory or a feeling of fogginess
- Inability to concentrate
- Problems sleeping

- Numbness or tingling of the arms or legs
- Arm, back, or shoulder discomfort
- Difficulty swallowing
- Lump in the throat

Frequently, these symptoms are frightening, discomforting, frustrating, annoying, and incapacitating. Certainly, they affect one's life style.

Expect symptoms to be more intense during emotional stress, when you are overly tired, after unaccustomed physical activities, during menopause, or during menstruation. It is not unusual for the symptoms to disappear spontaneously for months—even years—and reappear again.

Table 1-2 lists factors that increase the intensity or frequency of MVPS symptoms. These data were collected during the MVPS study, *Mitral Valve Prolapse Syndrome: Health Concerns, Role Function and Health Service Use.* Additional symptoms previously reported and compiled from data collected at the Mitral Valve Prolapse Program of Cincinnati (MVPPC), along with

TABLE 1-2. FACTORS THAT WORSEN MVPS SYMPTOMS (*N*=837)

	N	%
Emotional stress	653	78
Caffeine	564	67
Fatigue	538	64
Lack of sleep	525	63
Alcohol	263	31
Physical exertion	271	33
Menses	250	30
Foods	228	27
Exercise	188	23
Medications	155	19
Other	138	17
Tobacco	49	6
Marijuana	26	3
Cocaine	8	1

TABLE 1-3. ADDITIONAL FACTORS THAT WORSEN MVPS SYMPTOMS

• Unaccustomed physical activity
• Sweets, particularly on an empty stomach
• Being in a hot, dry environment
• Dehydration
• Flu, cold, or other illness
• Skipping meals
• Rushing around
• Lying on the left or right side
• Menses
• Menopause

responses to the questionnaire in the first and second editions of *Taking Control*, are give in Table 1-3.

Symptoms begin at any age. Most people, however, notice symptoms between the ages of 20 to 30. The exact cause likely relates to several factors and remains unclear. Often, MVPers who have been without symptoms become symptomatic after an illness, injury, pregnancy, or emotional stress such as a divorce. While symptoms occur more in females, many also occur in male MVPers. Frequently, chest pain, palpitations, fatigue, or anxiety attacks initially prompt them to seek medical help.

Many people with MVPS believe the more symptoms they have, the more severe is the prolapse—buckling back of the valve. This is *not* the case. In the mitral valve prolapse syndrome, there is no correlation between the degree of prolapse and the severity of the symptoms.

Metabolic-Neuroendocrine Abnormalities In MVPS

Research studies support the belief that certain physiological abnormalities may be responsible for MVPS symptoms. Not *everyone's* symptoms, however, are explained by these physiological alterations. The presence, degree, and type of involvement of the various physiological systems sometimes vary.

These physiological abnormalities include autonomic nervous system dysfunction, decreased intravascular blood volume, and renin–aldosterone regulation abnormality. These systems are interrelated, but are separately discussed.

Autonomic Nervous System Dysfunction

The body is under the constant control of the CNS—the central nervous system. This system is essential for our sense of well-being and our normal daily performance. The central nervous system controls and regulates in order to provide both stability and rapid, adaptive change to internal and external factors. Also, the central nervous system provides physiological, anticipatory adjustments. In other words, while certain body responses are under voluntary control, others are under involuntary control. For example, when you exercise, your heart rate normally increases to meet the demands of your body—an involuntary response. This response is controlled by the *autonomic nervous system*—the involuntary part of the CNS.

Two divisions make up the autonomic nervous system: the parasympathetic system (the decelerator) and the sympathetic system (the accelerator). In general, parasympathetic responses dominate when we are quiet, relaxed, or asleep, and sympathetic responses dominate when we are alert, excited, or engaged in muscular exercise. Note the following example that explains how these systems work.

You peacefully drive down the highway. Suddenly a Mack truck heads toward you. Your sympathetic nervous system—the accelerator—goes into action. It releases adrenalin. Your heart rate increases; your pupils dilate; and the blood supply to your muscles increases. Instantly, you have better braking action and can see better. You successfully avoid the truck. Now, to slow things down, the parasympathetic nervous system—the decelerator—takes over. It releases acetylcholine—a chemical substance—and you are ready to deal with the runaway truck.

Catecholamines are the chemical substances the sympathetic nervous system releases. Two major catecholamines are epinephrine (adrenalin) and norepinephrine. When these substances are released, they interact with cells in the blood vessels and in various organs. The part of the cell that responds to these chemicals is the receptor. A receptor is believed to be a site on the cell's surface where chemicals attach and initiate specific cellular processes.

Think of these receptors and chemicals as locks and keys—the lock is the receptor, and the chemical is the key. Whenever any key is turned, it determines a certain response. For example, epinephrine—depending upon which receptors are activated—causes blood vessels in skeletal muscle to narrow (vasoconstriction) or to enlarge (vasodilatation). Interaction of these chemicals with cells in the heart's electrical pacemaker increases the heart rate.

Instability, or imbalance, results when either the sympathetic system or the parasympathetic system are too active. This imbalance is referred to as *dysautonomia*—or autonomic dysfunction. People with MVPS sometimes have higher levels of catecholamines, alterations in catecholamine regulation, hypersensitivity to catecholamine stimulation and heightened parasympathetic responses. In other words, there is an increased number of locks, or keys, or both. These findings are believed to be responsible for a number of MVPS symptoms.

Dysautonomia—imbalance in the autonomic nervous system—is noted in people who have all the classic symptoms of MVPS, but have no objective findings of mitral valve prolapse. In other words, this person has no extra heart sounds or evidence of MVP on the echocardigoram. Their symptoms, however, are controllable with the non-drug treatments discussed in Chapter 4.

Renin–Aldosterone Regulation Abnormality

Research studies indicate some individuals with MVPS have alterations in how the body regulates water and sodium—salt, or the renin–aldosterone regulating system.

Aldosterone is the principal sodium-retaining steroid hormone—chemical substance. It maintains normal fluid balance and circulatory blood volume—fluid contained within the circulatory system. Normally, when blood volume decreases, as occurs with dehydration, the sympathetic nervous system activates and a special enzyme—renin—is secreted. This results in the release of aldosterone. Aldosterone causes sodium to be reabsorbed by the kidney and fluid to be retained. When blood volume is restored, renin secretion is suppressed.

In MVPS, there may be an abnormality in the regulation of this system. Studies show that after volume depletion caused by taking diuretics (water pills), renin activity and aldosterone release are reduced. Furthermore, renin activity is inappropriately low for the decreased circulating blood volume noted in people with MVPS.

Imagine this system as Larry-the-lock-controller on a dam. When the water level gets low—decreased circulating blood volume—Larry turns the wheel and closes the gates. The closed gates hold the water back, and cause a higher water level. Now, Larry becomes tired and doesn't close the wheel. What happens? The gates stay open, and the water level stays low. Likewise, this sometimes happens in MVPS—Larry lacks the energy to close the gates all the way.

Decreased Intravascular Volume

The volume of blood contained within the circulatory system is called the intravascular volume. It contains both plasma and the cellular elements of the blood. This blood volume is regulated through an intricate feedback mechanism. The integrity of this feedback mechanism is maintained by the kidneys, which regulate the blood volume either through an increase or decrease in urine excretion.

Studies indicate that people with MVPS sometimes have decreased plasma and intravascular volumes, which may be partly responsible for the lightheadedness, dizziness, and a forceful heart beat noted when first standing up.

Normally, whenever you stand from a lying position, cardiac output—amount of blood the heart pumps in a minute—increases. In some MVPers, however, cardiac output decreases when they first stand up. The decrease in cardiac output, along with a decrease in blood pressure and an increase in heart rate, causes feelings of lightheadedness, dizziness, and forceful heart pounding.

Likewise, this reduction in cardiac output—noted upon standing—may also continue during exercise. Coupled with the relatively high resting heart rate, it offers an explanation for the exercise intolerance and fatigue noted with MVPS.

The variations in intravascular volume and reduced renin–aldosterone activity help explain why some MVPers are very susceptible to volume depletion. These people note that their symptoms worsen after taking water pills or during crash dieting. Both cause water loss.

Magnesium Deficiency

Magnesium is an essential mineral required for multiple body functions. It is the fourth most common cation in the body and the second most common—after potassium—cation in cells. More than 300 enzymatic reactions depend on magnesium. This mineral affects the contractility of muscles, affects nerve conduction, and affects electrolyte balance. In the cardiovascular system magnesium influences both cardiac electrical and mechanical properties, and reactivity of blood vessels.

The majority of magnesium stores are in bone (60–65%), with the remainder in muscle (27%), soft tissues (19%), erythrocytes (0.5%), and in serum (0.3%). The reference interval for the total serum magnesium concentration is 0.75–0.96 mmol/L (1.8–2.3 mg/dL) and is the most common form for assessing Mg status. Since the serum contains only 0.3% of the total body Mg content and is not at equilibrium with other tissue pools of magnesium—with the exception of bone, it is not a good indicator of total body magnesium content. However, from a practical sense, clinical medicine uses the total serum magnesium concentration to assess magnesium status since this is essentially the only inexpensive, non-research-laboratory test offered by the clinical laboratory.

Evidence suggests that many features of MVP syndrome may be attributed to the physiologic effects of magnesium efficiency. Some people with MVPS have low blood levels of magnesium, particularly those with muscle cramps and migraines, two symptoms of magnesium deficiency. Other symptoms of magnesium deficiency include muscular weakness, lethargy, nausea, tremors, cardiac arrhythmias, and psychiatric abnormalities such as anxiety, depression, or nervous hyperexcitability. Interestingly, in the MVP Health Concerns study, we noted that MVPers who were more symptomatic had lower dietary intake of magnesium-rich foods.

Magnesium deficiency can be due to a reduced intake, reduced absorption, increased excretion, or redistribution of magnesium within the body. Large-scale dietary surveys reveal that the dietary intake of magnesium of most Americans falls below the recommended dietary allowance. Foods highest in magnesium—legumes, whole grains, and dark green leafy vegetables—are not major constituents of the average American diet. Also, reduced intake of magnesium occurs with dieting. Reduced absorption can occur with high saturated fat diets, or with the intake of substances such as dietary phosphates, which are very high in some sodas. Increased excretion can be caused by alcohol ingestion, diuretics, or excess sugar intake. Redistribution of magnesium occurs when levels of catecholamines are increased, as seen during psychological and physical stress. All of these factors increase magnesium requirements.

Selected References

ACC/AHA Guidelines for the Management of Patients with Valvular Heart Disease: A Report of the American College of Cardiology/American Heart Association Task Force on Practice Guidelines (Committee on Management of Patients With Valvular Heart Disease). 1998. *Journal of the American College of Cardiology* **32** (No. 5): 1486–1588.

Bashore, T., C. Grines, D. Utlak, J. Boudoulas & C. Wooley. 1985. Mitral valve prolapse: Postural exercise response reflects a volume disorder. *Journal of the American College of Cardiology* **5**: 504 (abstr).

Boudoulas, J. 1992. Mitral valve prolapse: Etiology, clinical presentation, and neuroendocrine function. *Journal of Heart Valve Disease* **1**: 175–188.

Coghlan, H. & G. Natello. 1991. Erythrocyte magnesium in symptomatic patients with primary mitral valve prolapse: Relationship to symptoms, mitral leaflet thickness, joint hypermobility and autonomic regulation. *Magnesium Trace Element* **92**: 205–214.

Coghlan, H., P. Phares, M. Cowley, D. Copley & T. James. 1979. Dysautonomia in mitral valve prolapse. *American Journal of Medicine* **67**: 236–244.

Elin, R. 1988. Magnesium metabolism in health and disease. *Disease of the Month* **34**: 161–219.

Ewing, D. 1988. Recent advances in the non-invasive investigation of diabetic autonomic neuropathy. *In* Autonomic Failure: A Textbook of Clinical Disorders of the Autonomic Nervous System. R. Bannister, Ed., pp. 667–689. Oxford University Press. Oxford.

Fontana, M., C. Wooley, R. Leighton & R. Lewis. 1975. Postural changes in left ventricular and mitral valvular dynamics in the systolic click-late systolic murmur syndrome. Circulation **51:** 165–173.

Freed, L., J.S.J. Acierno, D. Dai, M. Leyne, J. Marshall, F. Nesta *et al.* 2003. A locus for autosomal dominant mitral valve prolapse on chromosome 11p15.4. *American Journal of Human Genetics* **72**(6): 1551–1559.

Gaffney, F., & C. Blomqvist. 1988. Mitral valve prolapse and autonomic nervous system dysfunction: A pathophysiological link. *In* Mitral Valve Prolapse and the Mitral Valve Prolapse Syndrome. H. Boudoulas & C. Wooley, Eds., pp. 427–443. Futura Publishing Co. New York.

Galland, L., S. Baker & R. McLellan. 1986. Magnesium deficiency in the pathogenesis of mitral valve prolapse. *Magnesium* **5:** 165–174.

Halpern, M, & J. Durlach, Eds. 1985. Magnesium Deficiency: Physiopathology and Treatment Implications. First European Congress on Magnesium, Lisbon, October 6–8, 1983. Karger. New York.

Hayek, E. & B. Griffin. 2002. Mitral valve prolapse: old beliefs yield to new knowledge. *Cleveland Clinic Journal of Medicine* **69**(11): 889–896.

Hayek, E., C. Gring & B.P. Griffin. 2005. Mitral valve prolapse. Lancet **365** (9458), 507–518.

Jeresaty, R. 1979. Mitral Valve Prolapse. Raven Press. New York.

Kitlinski, M., W. Piwowarska, E. Konduracka, D. Mroczek-Czernecka & J. Nessler. 1999. Variability of heart auscultation in patients with mitral valve prolapse. *Przeglad Lekarski* **56:** 783-786.

Kitlinski, M., M. Stepniewski, J. Nessler, E. Konduracka, K. Solarska, W. Piwowarska & L. Erhardt. 2004. Is magnesiuim deficit in lymphocytes a part of the mitral valve prolapse syndrome? *Magnesium Research* **17:** 39–45.

Kolibash, A. 1988. Natural history of mitral valve prolapse. *In* Mitral Valve Prolapse and the Mitral Valve Prolapse Syndrome. H. Boudoulas & C. Wooley, Eds., pp. 257–274. Futura Publishing Co. New York.

Lowenstein, F.W. & Stanton, F. 1986. Serum magnesium levels in the United States, 1971–1974. *Journal of the American College of Nutrition* **5**(4): 399–414.

Nascimento, R., A. Freitas, F. Teixeira, *et al.* 1997. *American Journal of Cardiology* **79**(2): 226–227.

Practice Guideline for the Treatment of Patients with Borderline Personality Disorder. October, 2001. The American Psychiatric Association. Available at www.psych.org.Society.

Rude, R. 1989. Physiology of magnesium metabolism and the important role of magnesium in potassium deficiency. *American Journal of Cardiology* **63**: 31G–43G.

Schondorf, R. & P.A. Low. 1993. Idiopathic postural orthostatic tachycardia syndrome: an attenuated form of acute pan-dysdautonomia? Neurology **43**: 132–137.

Scordo, K. 2004. Symptom control for mitral valve prolapse. *The Clinical Advisor* : 37–41.

Scordo, K. 2005. Mitral valve prolapse syndrome: health concerns, symptoms and treatments. *Western Journal of Nursing Research* **27**(4): 390–405.

Seeing, M. 1989. Cardiovascular consequences of magnesium deficiency and loss: Pathogenesis, prevalence and manifestations-magnesium and chloride loss in refractory potassium repletion. *American Journal of Cardiology* **63**: 4G–22G.

Sobo, S. 1999. Mood stabilizers and mood swings: In search of a definition. *Psychiatric Times* **16**: 36–42.

2

Diagnosing Mitral Valve Prolapse

Being diagnosed with MVP can be problematic. Some of the symptoms associated with MVPS may be present in a variety of other clinical conditions. Therefore, people often report that MVP was not their initial diagnosis. Many MVPers consulted several physicians and received conflicting diagnoses as listed below:

- hypoglycemia—low blood sugar
- chronic fatigue syndrome
- hypothyroidism; hyperthyroidism
- Ménière's disease—inner ear problem
- anxiety disorder
- multiple sclerosis
- fibromyalgia
- esophagitis

In making the diagnosis of MVP, the practitioner considers a variety of factors. These include your present symptoms, past history, family history, results of physical examination, and diagnostic tests.

A key factor in diagnosing mitral valve prolapse is auscultation (listening to) of the heart. The presence of a click with or without a systolic murmur is characteristic of MVP. The click is an extra heart sound caused by the tensing of the chords that facilitate the opening and closing of the valve. A systolic murmur is a sound that occurs during the heart's contraction when a small amount of blood flows backward—through a partially opened mitral valve—into the left atrium.

Changes in posture may alter the characteristics of the click and murmur. In fact, the click and/or murmur may only be heard when standing, or when lying on your left side. Your practitioner, therefore, may listen to your heart when you are squatting, standing, lying down, or lying on your left side. In addition, MVP is a very dynamic syndrome and the click or

**MOST COMMON SYMPTOMS
FOR SEEKING ASSISTANCE OF A PHYSICIAN***

- Palpitations, extra beats, irregular heartbeat, pounding heart, racing heart, skipped beats, rapid pulse, heart fluttering
- Chest pain, chest tightness
- Lightheadedness, dizziness, almost passing out
- Fatigue, weakness
- Anxiety/panic attacks
- Shortness of breath
- Headaches

*Data from *Taking Control* questionnaire.

murmur may not always be heard. People commonly say, "Sometimes my physician hears the murmur, and sometimes he doesn't." If you take beta blockers or tranquilizers, or are well hydrated, the click or murmur—or both—may be inaudible.

The echocardiogram can be used to confirm the diagnosis. This ultrasound examination of the heart consists of an M-mode—or ice-pick view—of the heart along with a two dimensional (2D) view. This test gives information about the mitral valve, the other valves, the thickness of the walls of the heart, the size of the heart's chambers, and how well the heart contracts. Color Doppler shows the presence and degree of mitral regurgitation—or backward blood flow. MVP is diagnosed when one or both mitral leaflets exhibit at least 2 millimeters of posterior displacement (buckling back) into the left atrium. Consideration is also given to structural changes such as leaflet thickening and elongation of the chords. It is possible, however, to have MVP and not see it on the echocardiogram. Conversely, it is possible to see MVP on the echo and not have the classic auscultatory findings.

To screen for possible coronary artery disease, a graded exercise stress test is done. Prior to the start of a stress test, the technician places foam-filled disks on your chest. The disks connect to wires. The wires connect to a heart monitor. The monitor records your heart's electrical activity. As you walk on the treadmill, the speed and grade (height) of the treadmill increase at specified times. (A bicycle may be used in place of the treadmill.) The technician monitors your blood pressure before, during, and after the test. The test provides information about your level of cardiovascular fitness, your blood pressure response to exercise, and any exercise-induced abnormalities in heart rhythm. Also, this test may show EKG changes that *suggest* ischemia—lack of oxygen to a portion of the heart muscle. This may, however, be a false-positive result.

At times, MVPers have false-positive results on exercise stress tests that occur with or without chest pain. In other words, there are changes on the EKG similar to those seen with ischemic coronary artery disease, but the person does not have cardiac, coronary, or artery disease. This is particularly common in woman. In this situation, a test that combines a graded exercise stress test with the injection of a radioisotope provides further diagnostic information. Exercise Tc^{99m}Cardiolite, thallium-201, or Myoview™ are examples.

When these radioisotopes are injected, they normally distribute throughout the heart muscle. The amount of the isotope the heart muscle takes up is directly related to its blood flow. If a coronary artery is narrowed or blocked, the isotope doesn't distribute to the area supplied by this artery. Therefore, when pictures of the heart are taken, a cold spot or dark area shows on the film. At a later time, the pictures are repeated. If the cold spot no longer shows, it suggests a narrowing of a coronary artery. If the cold spot remains, it suggests a previous heart attack.

To decrease the degree of false-positive results, the treadmill test can be combined with a 2D echocardiogram and is called an exercise stress echocardiogram, or simply a stress echo. This test evaluates heart function by combining an exercise (stress) test with an echocardiogram. A stress echocardiogram provides images of the heart both before (sometimes during) and immediately following exercise. How the heart responds to exercise is evaluated by comparing images of the heart at rest with images of the heart during and/or after exercise. Decreased movement of a section of the heart wall with exercise suggests myocardial (heart muscle) ischemia.

An additional heart test is electron-beam computed tomography (EBCT)—also known as ultra-fast CT. This test, however, is usually reserved to screen high-risk asymptomatic persons for the development of coronary artery disease (CAD), or used to determine the presence of CAD in symptomatic people. EBCT is a highly sensitive technique that detects calcium deposits in the coronary arteries. Calcium in the coronary arteries indicates atherosclerosis—the buildup of plaques that can lead to a heart attack. The amount of coronary calcium is related to the extent of coronary plaque disease. This test takes a few minutes and requires you to lie face up on an examination table under a CT scanner. An electron beam generates X-rays (four times as strong as a simple chest X-ray) that pass through your body. Technicians identify the calcium deposits in the images, and then use a computer program to derive a coronary artery calcium score that reflects the total calcium "load" in the coronary arteries. Scores of 0 to 10 reflect arteries largely free from coronary plaque (minimal coronary calcification). Scores of 11 to 400 indicate mild to moderate plaque buildup; scores above 400 indicate extensive plaque. Studies have shown that people with higher calcium scores are at greater risk for heart attacks and strokes than those with very low scores. A major limitation of EBCT, however, is its inability to reliably identify the "vulnerable plaque"—or the soft, unstable plaque in the artery wall that breaks open and causes the formation of an artery-plugging blood clot. Be aware that the cost of the test ranges from $100 to $600 and is usually *not* covered by insurance companies.

Sometimes, a heart catheterization may be needed This involves injecting small amounts of dye into the coronary arteries via a catheter or small hollow tube. A physician usually recommends this for any number of reasons. Is the person over 40? Does he have a strong family history of heart disease or other cardiac risk factors? Are there suspicious symptoms of coronary artery disease? Was the exercise nuclear study abnormal? Are the calcium scores high?

After you have been diagnosed with MVP, the follow-up with your physician is similar to others without MVP, that is, annual physical examination. Some physicians recommend repeat echocardiograms every few years to note changes in the mitral valve structure, the chamber sizes, the wall thickness, and the heart muscle's contractions. Consult your physician if your symptoms change, or if you are unsure whether they relate to MVPS.

The presence and degree of dysautonomia is determined by autonomic testing. This involves the use of noninvasive, cardiovascular reflex tests. A noninvasive test does not require any needle punctures, incisions, or insertion of instruments. These reflex tests include:

1. The heart rate response to a simulated Valsalva maneuver—with your nose closed, blowing into a mouthpiece at a certain pressure.

2. Deep breathing.
3. Blood pressure and heart rate responses to standing or with head up on a tilt table.
4. Sustained handgrip—holding a special handgrip device.

There are normal responses to these tests. Sometimes the test is repeated and results compared to determine the efficacy of certain treatment interventions. Furthermore, your level of plasma catecholamines can be determined. This blood test measures levels of epinephrine and norepinephrine.

Summary

MVPS, a common clinical condition, affects millions of people throughout the world. Only within the past decade have researchers identified a physiologic basis for its symptoms.

Previously—as correspondence from MVPers shows—many have endured one misdiagnosis after another until someone truly believed—"it's *not* all in your head."

Although definitive methods for long-term treatment of MVPS are still under study, don't give up. Follow the recommendations discussed in this book. Use this knowledge to change the quality of your life. TAKE CONTROL.

Selected References

Agency for Healthcare Research and Quality. Results of systematic review of research on diagnosis and treatment of coronary heart disease in women. Evidence Report/ Technology Assessment Number 80. U.S. Department of Health and Human Services, Public Health Services. AHRQ Pub. No. 03-E034, May 2003.

Boudoulas, J. & C. Wooley. 1988. Mitral valve prolapse: Clinical presentation and diagnostic evaluation. *In* Mitral Valve Prolapse and the Mitral Valve Prolapse Syndrome, H. Boudoulas & C. Wooley, Eds. pp. 299–330. Futura Publishing Co. New York.

DeCara, J. 2003. Noninvasive cardiac testing in women. *JAMWA* **58:** 254–263.

Kasper, D.L. *et al.* Eds. 2005. Harrison's Principles of Internal Medicine. 16th ed. McGraw-Hill. New York.

Kwok, Y., C. Kim, D. Grady, *et al.* 1999. Meta-analysis of exercise testing to detect coronary artery disease in women. *American Journal of Cardiology* **83:** 660–666.

Gibbons, R., J. Abrams, K. Chatterjee, *et al.* 1997. A report of the American College of Cardiology/American Heart Association Task Force on Practice Guidelines (Committee on Exercise Testing). *Journal of the American College of Cardiology* **30:** 260–315.

Mieres, J., L. Shaw, R. Hendel, *et al.* 2003. Consensus statement: American Society of Nuclear Cardiology: Task force on women and coronary artery disease—The role of myocardial perfusion imaging in the clinical evaluation of coronary artery disease in women. *Journal of Nuclear Cardiology* **10:** 95–101.

Manning, W., M. Stuber, P. Danias, R. Botnar, S. Yeon & F. Aepfelbacher. 2002. Coronary magnetic resonance imaging. *Current Problems in Cardiology* **27:** 275–333.

Modena, M.G., A. Nuzzo & R. Rossi. 2003. Gender differences in diagnostic procedures. *Italian Heart Journal* **4:** 518–521.

Scordo, K. 2005. Non-invasive diagnosis of coronary artery disease in women. *Journal of Cardiovascular Nursing* **20:** 420–426.

3

People with MVPS
Share Their Experiences

The universe is made of stories, not of atoms.
MURIEL RUKEYSER, 1980

According to your many letters, e-mails, and responses to the questionnaire in the first and second editions of *Taking Control*, this chapter was by far the most popular. Comments such as these were common: "I'm so glad to hear I'm not alone." "That sounds just like me." "I really enjoyed reading what others did to control their symptoms."

In the Fall of 1992, because of these comments, the feature "Tell It Like It Is" began in *Network*, the former newsletter of the MVP Program of Cincinnati. This column encouraged people to share their experiences. Letters poured in from all over the world. These stories were incorporated into the first two editions of the book; some remain in this edition. A recent call for MVPS stories provided additional content for this chapter. Of interest is that 56% of participants in the MVPS Health Concerns study wrote comments ranging from a few sentences to seven typed pages. Examples of these comments are: "My cardiologist said to go home and don't think about it [the symptoms];" "Fear is a problem I have to work with. Fear of a panic attack. Symptoms cause me to fear that I will get worse and have to go to the emergency room;" "These symptoms have limited my joys in life—I fear exercise and medications. I feel so hopeless;" "When I was diagnosed with MVP, my physician at the time did not explain just what it was or how it would or would not have an impact on my life. I admit, I was scared;" "Just going on vacation to another country gave me a feeling of panic. I WANT TO GO HOME! All the time thinking what if something happens? Where would I go—I don't want to meet strange doctors! I can't enjoy my vacations because of these feelings of panic. I fear these skipped beats will result in a total disaster or just sudden death. It's terrifying.

Stories range from those who, on the first visit, were correctly diagnosed with MVPS to those who, after *dozens* of visits to various physicians, were diagnosed with MVPS. Many say their symptoms interfere with activities of daily living, with family relations, and with work relations. Frequently, individuals share fears experienced before they were correctly diagnosed—fears of not knowing what was going on and why they had symptoms. Some were told, "It's all in you head," and believed they were going crazy. Others became unsettled when told, "You have MVP and chest pain ... don't worry about it."

As you read the following accounts from real people with MVPS, you may identify with certain aspects of their stories. Some of these individuals either completed the program or attended the educational seminars—others didn't. Some were diagnosed recently—others were diagnosed years ago. In several of the following accounts, note two recurring themes: "initial distress," noted prior to diagnosis, and "later comfortableness," noted after diagnosis and explanations.

Vanessa

"I am 44 years old with two children 13 and 16 and have been suffering with MVPS for 12 years. Only for the last four months have I actually known what was causing my endless, sometimes debilitating, symptoms.

"My symptoms started with full-blown panic attacks shortly after the birth of my second child. There were the emergency room visits, the inability to drive, and general anxiety for years. I learned to live with it and tried my best to manage it. While in the hospital with the first panic attack I was diagnosed with mitral valve prolapse. I was told it was not a big deal and not to worry about it. Over the years my symptoms mutated into many different symptoms. I thought nothing could be worse than a panic attack, but I soon discovered there was. At least I knew panic attacks would eventually go away. These new symptoms were defining my life in a bad way. I have had very severe nausea that would put me in bed for a week at a time. I had diarrhea, numbness in hands, feet and face, mood swings, chest pains, heart palpitations, night sweats, shaking inside, depression, fatigue, dry mouth, anxiety, and insomnia. I would go to the hospital when it got bad and I had to have fluids because I was dehydrated. I canceled trips, missed school functions and really felt alone and helpless.

"My family was very supportive and helpful. My husband was supportive but after all of these years of me 'not feeling well' and every medical test was negative; I think he actually thought I was making it up. After being diagnosed I sometimes think he doesn't recognize my condition as being real. Over the years he has always been there during a panic attack and helped me through, but it is hard for a person who feels well all of the time to understand the daily struggle this syndrome causes.

> After twelve years it took ME to figure out what was wrong with me!

"To find out what was wrong, I've been to seven different physicians, including a psychologist. I have been diagnosed with panic disorder, irritable bowel syndrome, stomach ulcers and mitral valve prolapse. I have a pharmacy full of medications. I have been told that nothing physically was wrong with me, that it could quite possibly be in my head. I have been put on birth control pills, tried to go 'organic' and have been told by my internist there was simply nothing else he could do.

"I've learned that caffeine makes my heart beat harder and faster, and thus avoid all caffeinated beverages. I also discovered that I am very sensitive to MSG (monosodium glutamate). This makes me very ill with severe heart palpitations; sometimes I would be confined to bed with nausea for days after ingesting MSG.

"Finally, after years of begging physicians to help me and praying for an answer, I read one sentence in a book that I think helped to save me from the hell I was living. Then, while I watched the Oprah show, I saw physician who wrote a book called *The Manual of You.* I immediately ordered it. I thought if I learned more about my body I might be able to figure out what was wrong with me and help myself—no one else could. In the chapter about your heart, I read that mitral valve prolapse goes hand in hand with panic attacks in young women. FINALLY, a light bulb went off. No doctor ever suggested that prolapse had anything to do with my symptoms. Not one doctor I saw ever suggested that the mitral valve could be involved. After twelve years it took ME to figure out what was wrong with me!

"I went online and cried when I read that there were actually other people out there in the world like me. A LOT of other people. I went online to MVPSupport.com and couldn't believe it. There was actually a name for what I had, I wasn't crazy and maybe, just maybe I could find someone to help me now. I was up half the night reading the support boards.

"I immediately went on 500 mg of magnesium a day and began forcing fluids. I was a big water drinker before but now I was making sure I got the 64–80 oz of water in a day. Just these two small adjustments were slowly helping with my general feeling and it noticeably helped my fatigue.

"The next day I called and made an appointment at The Mitral Valve Prolapse/Dysautonomia Center in Birmingham, Alabama. I had a tilt table test, a stress test, blood tests and more. This was a very emotional experience. I could not believe I was sitting in front of physician who believed me and understood what I had lived through. I was told I had enough adrenaline in my body for six people. I learned about low blood volume, malfunction of the autonomic nervous system and about the importance of exercise and diet. I was prescribed Zebata®, a beta blocker, Lexapro® (for anxiety), and Klonopin® (for sleep).

"I am presently exercising, taking 250 mg of magnesium in the morning, drinking plenty of water, taking the Zebata and the Klonopin. My quality of life is slowly improving. I still have setbacks and I get through them by telling myself it is better than it was. Since I have started on my medication, the magnesium, the water, no caffeine, magnesium, and exercising regularly, I think there may be an end in sight. The most comforting thing when I am not feeling well is I have a physical explanation to my symptoms. It makes you feel better knowing that there has actually been a diagnosis and that there are reasons why my face is numb, why I am dizzy and disconnected, why my heart is beating fast and hard. If I am dizzy and numb I drink, drink, drink or eat a pretzel or a salty snack to hold the water. It usually helps. I still have bad days, especially around my period, but I try to get through them knowing there are better days ahead.

"This is a life-altering syndrome. I have lived with MVP for twelve years not knowing what is was. Hopefully now with the knowledge and education I have received from books and my experience in Alabama, my next twelve years will be brighter!"

Tricia

"I am a 31-year-old female who has had strange health problems since I was 16. As a child, I was healthy, but at age 16, I started to have major allergies, fatigue, and very low energy—in fact, I gained 50 pounds. I felt weak, faint and was frequently sick. Illness would incapacitate me for weeks at a time. At 18, I had a near fainting episode. I went blind and almost deaf for a matter of minutes and felt as if I would die. My heart was pounding, but I was able to speak throughout the experience. I had a diving accident that year and attributed the experience to a possible neck injury. Through my early 20's I was frequently ill and thus missed lots of work. I never had any energy. Medications adversely affected me. Weather changes made me feel as if I had the flu. In other words, I was miserable. At age 25, I because pregnant. I was extremely sick—no energy, nausea for nine months. During this time I noted palpitations, especially after I ate. Every symptom I had because worse. Despite my symptoms, all my blood tests were normal. After the birth of my son, I decided that I could not physically handle another pregnancy."

> **All in all, this experience has been life altering—I am so glad to find out that I am not crazy.**

"I have always had a high stress life. I am a high school English teacher and was the music minister in my church and director of women's ministry. I became a senior sales director in Mary Kay the next year and my stress level went way up. I started getting sick and rundown even more. Three years later, I resigned and sent back my car. My days were so unpredictable. Some days I would feel almost normal, and then the next morning I would not be able to get out of bed. Still no one knew what was wrong with me. I thought I was going crazy! At 29, I started getting sick every month. After I would lead the music at church I would get sick. Finally, an ear, nose and throat physician figured out that my tonsils were awful. I was put on steroids. After a few weeks on the medication, I thought I was going to die. I gained weight, felt awful, and had heart palpitations once again. Two months later, I underwent a tonsillectomy. I started having terrible TMJ problems that were misdiagnosed by my family doctor as ear infections. I was on antibiotics for a while, which my body didn't handle well. Finally, my ENT doctor realized that I had TMJ. The swelling in my face and ear felt like horrible ear infections. I was put on medication with some relief. The medicine, however, gave me chest tightness, some palpitations.

"I then started seeing a chiropractor, who helped me more that anyone. In addition to adjustments, he put me on some natural substances that made me feel much better. I started having more good days and losing weight. That was last year. In January of this year, I got so run down and weak that I had to quit my job. I found out in February that I was pregnant. Once again, my symptoms began: heart palpitations, chest tightness, severe fatigue and shortness of breath. My doctor thought I might have a thyroid problem—she sent me to a perinatal and fertility specialist who told me that I didn't have a thyroid problem; these were pregnancy symptoms. I was so disappointed that I didn't have a thyroid problem I cried. I was then diagnosed with depression. My internist sent me to a cardiologist who performed several tests and found nothing wrong with my heart. Another thyroid test and now to an endocrinologist. His nurse mentioned a completely benign condition called mitral valve prolapse, but told me it was nothing. The endocrinologist was equally helpful. She said my thyroid was off due to pregnancy and that I was having panic attacks and depression. I told her and the other physicians that I was pretty sure that I was emotionally healthy. It was the physicians who were making me depressed! I went home completely exhausted. Every visit to a new doctor meant another 2–4 weeks of waiting and hoping for an answer only to be let down every time. During this time, I got some type of head cold for the second time since pregnancy. I was so sick. Finally, I took my doctor's advice and took one Sudafed. I thought I was going to have a heart attack and ended up in the emergency room. They too could find nothing except a low iron level. A few days later, I went to see one of the midwives in my doctor's office. She listened to me as I described my symptoms and shared with me that she had similar symptoms. She told me that she had a mitral valve prolapse and hypoglycemia. I then remembered what the nurse had told me about my MVP. This was the beginning to the answer. From that point on, I researched everything that I could find. I am almost positive that I have an autonomic nervous system imbalance. I have found information on the magnesium connection and am taking that now. I'm still pregnant and having symptoms, but they have lessened. I now drink lots of water, eat more protein, and avoid caffeine and sugar. This does help alleviate most of my palpitations. Weather changes continue to affect me. The day before I get irritable and fatigued, during the change, I ache, and at times have a low-grade temperature and feel pressure in my body.

"My father has similar symptoms and has been in the hospital with feelings of a heart attack. The doctors found that his heart was beating extremely fast, but they could not figure why. They gave him some medication to slow it down. He has these attacks when he is extremely stressed. They don't happen very often. He also gets sick easily and worn down and is affected by weather changes. My sister is turning 18 this year, and she started having occasional mild heart palpitations. My paternal grandfather recently told my dad that he had the same heart symptoms that my dad does. And now my paternal aunt is in the hospital having major tests run for heart attack–type symptoms or perhaps an arrhythmia. During her previous ER visit, with similar symptoms, she was told that a heart attack is very unlikely. All in all, this experience has been life-altering—I am so glad to find out that I am not crazy."

Lorelei

"It had been a particularly stressful few weeks. My nine-month-old son had just started walking—getting into everything he shouldn't. Then, after living with my mother-in-law for quite some time, my husband and I moved into our first apartment. After being a stay-at-home mom, I was hired for a job—a job for which I was inexperienced. To complicate matters, our finances weren't the best. After not driving for five years, I purchased a car to make the 45-minute journey to my new job. Now I needed a baby-sitter—a position hard to fill. In such a short time, my life dramatically changed. I was 23 years young, healthy, and I felt I could handle any situation. Change was for the better—right? And we needed the additional income. So why did I feel so stressed?

"A short time later, everything came to a head. I had spent the day alone with my son. When I put him down for the night, I was exhausted. In fact, it was such a busy day, I forgot to eat. I finished putting away toys, cleaning the kitchen, washing clothes and taking out the trash. At about midnight, I awoke from sleep when I heard my husband return from work. My full bladder led me to the bathroom. As I stumbled back to bed, I remember feeling extremely lightheaded. Everything was spinning around me. As I lay in bed, I felt worse. I thought perhaps I'm dehydrated and some water will help. That did help a bit, but within an hour, my head continued to swim. I began to uncontrollably shake—in fact, I had diarrhea. I was nervous. What's happening? I called my physician. 'You can't faint when you're lying down—just go back to bed and relax,' was his response. I felt like I was on death's doorstep. After two hours, I wasn't any better and headed for the emergency room. I was told there was nothing wrong—perhaps I was under unusual stress. Then I remembered all the recent changes in my life. Yes, they're probably right—it's all in my head. My diagnosis was an anxiety attack for which I was given a prescription for an antihistamine derivative to help me sleep.

"In the days that followed, I slowly sank into hell. Every day a new symptom would appear—insomnia, fatigue, panic attacks, migraine headaches, chronic diarrhea, chest pains, and tingling and numbness in my fingers. These symptoms led me to my physician's office. Each time, I was tested for something new—diabetes, hypoglycemia, and an overactive thyroid—all with normal results. The only finding was a a slight decrease in my iron level. I was prescribed Zantac to control all the acid my stomach was producing, and Xanax and then Ativan to calm me down, and finally Zoloft to control my depression. Never had I been on so many medications at once! I was determined not to rely on drugs for the rest of my life. Appointments were to be made for upper G.I. and lower G.I. tests. I could feel myself becoming a hypochondriac, and I hated it! I lost about twenty pounds that summer, along with most of my sanity.

"That was my existence for three months. Even so, I began my new job and really enjoyed the demanding work. I was a mortgage company's settlement officer and, although extremely stressful, it was exciting. I got used to taking 'Imodium A-D breaks' every day. In fact, I thought about buying stock in the company. When I got home at night, I fed my baby, played with him for a couple of hours before he went to bed, did laundry and dishes, cleaned the house, ate a quick dinner, and fell into bed. I accepted what the physicians were telling me, that it was all in my head.

> I accepted what the physicians were telling me, that it was all in my head.

"As time progressed, the symptoms became worse. To regain control, I was advised to seek psychiatric counseling. I began to see a private counselor—just talking about my feelings helped. I still didn't feel like I belonged there, so I only went for a few months. A short while later, I called her to let her know I was about to admit myself to the psychiatric unit of the local hospital—I thought I was having a nervous breakdown. That morning I couldn't get dressed. I just sat on the couch shivering—as if it was 30 degrees. I wondered how I could manage to survive. I was crying, and felt like I was losing my mind. She laughed and told me that if I had the presence of mind to call her and tell her I was having a nervous breakdown, then she was positive that I was not. That made me feel better, but I was still shaking horribly and having non-stop diarrhea. My head was spinning out of control, and I felt like an emotional wreck! When I got to the hospital, they had me speak to a psychiatric nurse who told me, after we talked at length, that she believed I was not having a breakdown or going crazy. She began to tell me the most interesting story about her mother, who had had similar symptoms, and was diagnosed with mitral valve prolapse (MVP).

"Mitral valve prolapse? I recognized the name of the genetic condition. I knew that's what my grandmother had. Later I found out that at least five of my relatives also have MVP. I told the physician my previous doctor heard a heart murmur when I was sixteen, but there was no further mention since then. I had an echocardiogram of my heart. That confirmed by diagnosis: mitral valve prolapse. To check for extra beats, I wore a 24-hour Holter monitor. I was given a prescription for Inderal and sent home. I was to follow up yearly with a cardiologist and take prophylactic antibiotics before dental procedures. I finally had a name for what was ruining my life. My problem was I didn't fully understand how a heart condition could cause all the weird symptoms. I also didn't understand why, if I was born with MVP, it took this long for me to find out I had it. Could it really be possible that MVP was the culprit? It was hard to believe, especially since for the past three months I was led to believe it was all in my head. I recalled a few episodes of fainting spells I'd had since a child, my low exercise tolerance, and occasional palpitations. Was it possible that MVP was the cause? I made an appointment with a cardiologist and waited for the opportunity to get some answers to my questions.

"Unfortunately, the cardiologist didn't have any helpful answers. I was told: It's possible that the symptoms are related, but they aren't life-threatening and you shouldn't worry about dying or getting ill or anything. Easy for him to say. I was beginning to believe that I made no progress. Was MVP causing my symptoms, or not? The answer had to be clear-cut, and I was determined to find my answer. I went home with the pamphlet called "Mitral Valve Prolapse—A Slight Difference in a Healthy Heart" [Krames Communications, 1988] and thoroughly read it . It didn't take long to realize that according to this information, the only problem I might ever have is palpitations now and then.

"About six months later, I read an article in a fitness magazine about a lady who had been diagnosed with MVP and who had found a support group through a diagnosis and treatment center in Alabama. I blinked my eyes in disbelief and read the whole article again. There was actually a whole center devoted to diagnosis and treatment of MVP? I had to find out more. I called the operator to get the area code for the city and state where the center was located, then I called information in that state and asked for the center's phone number: no listing. I had to get a hold of this center! Another six months went by, and my symptoms were still bothering me a great deal. I went through all my papers looking for the same magazine article I had read the past winter—and I finally found it. I sat staring at it in frustration, and then realized that the woman who had written it had listed the city and state where she lived—along with her last name. Why hadn't this occurred to me before? I couldn't believe my luck! I called information again and they gave me her number. I was shaking as I dialed it, what if she was really upset that I was bothering her like this? This was invasion of privacy in a big way. I tried to calm down by telling myself that if she hadn't wanted anyone to get this information, she wouldn't have allowed all of it to be printed in the first place. Still, I was nervous. As it turned out I was only able to talk to her answering machine anyway. I left my phone number and the reason I was calling, and asked her to please call me back. Then about two weeks went by. I figured that she must have really been upset that some stranger was calling her and that she didn't want to call me back—I definitely wasn't about to call her again. Then one day in the middle of the afternoon, she called. It was wonderful to speak to someone who had the same condition that I did. I felt like I wasn't alone after all. She gave me the phone number I needed (it turned out that I hadn't been giving the full name of the center and that's why I couldn't get the number through Information) and said that she would have called sooner but that she had been on vacation. After thanking her for calling, I immediately called the center and asked them to please find a support group for me in my area. The best they could do was to tell me of one that was in a neighboring state—an hour's drive away. I didn't care, as long as I could talk to other people about what I was going through, and to find out if anyone else was suffering like I was. I called the leader of the group who told me that the support group was just forming and the first meeting would be in two months—and that she would send me a book about MVP right away.

"When I received the book, I looked at the front cover and started crying. I sat down on the floor and just sobbed because

I felt so relieved ... right there, in bold letters, was a list of all the symptoms I had been suffering from! I felt so completely validated. It was a turning point in my life. I read the book from cover to cover right then and there—and that night, I read it again. The book spoke of 'mitral valve prolapse syndrome,' not simply mitral valve prolapse. Could there be a difference between the two? And if so, which did I have? Although it wasn't always easy, I began to try re-training my thoughts so that I wouldn't automatically think that I was going crazy when I started to feel the old feelings of anxiety, and all the symptoms that went along with it. Now the time had come to get my hands on every piece of information that there was on mitral valve prolapse syndrome (MVPS), and to work on understanding the difference between it and MVP—if there was any.'

"This affected my so much that I wrote a book, *Mitral Valve Prolapse Syndrome: A Patient's Perspective*. My goal is relay information I learned about how to cope with MVPS—my tricks and tips on how to control the symptoms, advice for family and friends of those diagnosed, advice on how to change your lifestyle to reduce the occurrence of symptoms, specific information regarding how to handle panic and anxiety attacks, and to reassure all of you—through personal stories—that you are not alone. I also have a website. I hope you'll visit me at: http://www.MVPSupport.com."

Marci

"My story is rather tame compared to some that I have come upon. My symptoms started about four years ago, when I was 33 years of age and after a rather stressful year. I began blacking out when standing up from a lying position. My physician knew right away what it was, just from the description of this symptom and a quick listen to my heart, and scheduled me for an echocardiogram, which confirmed that I had MVP with regurgitation. I was irritated with the diagnosis because I have always been healthy, regularly exercised, ate fairly well, got adequate rest, and maintained my weight. At least I knew right then that I wasn't crazy.

"I began to get very emotional and I was so sure that I was pregnant because of the nausea, headaches, etc. My husband was very puzzled about my emotional issues; I was always crying and moody and uninterested in everyday things. He also worried when I complained of chest pain. I began reading everything I could about the condition. I realized that I have the typical physical features described in the studies: tall, thin with long limbs, and slight scoliosis. Although I was relieved that it is not a degenerative condition, I still needed to find a way to relieve the symptoms. It seemed little was known about what caused the symptoms, let alone what would alleviate them. I began seeing how lucky I was to have received a quick diagnosis—many people have suffered a long time before being diagnosed. There are also plenty of people out there who are experiencing life-altering symptoms on a daily basis. I was determined not to end up this way.

> I've realized that it is definitely worth it to take the time to take care of myself.

"By chance, I decided to give in to the pleas of my own mother to take calcium everyday. I began taking calcium and decided to take a multi-vitamin along with it. Taking daily vitamins relieved my symptoms tremendously! (Thank you, Mom!) I have since read that MVPers tend to have certain vitamin/mineral deficiencies, so I take them faithfully every day.

"I still have one or two dominant symptoms. These occur mainly during extreme temperatures, when I'm tired or stressed. They mostly consist of headaches, nausea, "lump in the throat" feeling, chest/neck/arm pain, shortness of breath, 'awareness of the heart,' cold hands and feet, etc. Sometimes there are feelings and sensations that are indescribable. Occasionally, my bottom teeth feel like super-cold water is passing through them or my chest feels completely empty or a bad taste will fill my mouth. Waking up in the middle of the night not knowing where I am or thinking people or things are in the room is the worst! But these symptoms are all bearable. I have never had a panic attack or paranoia or extreme fatigue or depression or anything else that disrupts my life. I firmly believe this is due to the fact that I am progressively eating better, taking vitamins, getting enough sleep and, although I can't exercise as much, I still do it regularly. I've realized that it is definitely worth it to take the time to take care of myself. I believe that the power of proper maintenance of the mind and body is underestimated when it comes to any medical ailment. I have made the choice not to be on medication. I plan on taking care of myself for the rest of my life and staying positive for the sake of my family. I am just very thankful that physicians and researchers are becoming more aware and knowledgeable of the causes and symptoms. I am also thankful for those devoting their lives to research and improving the quality of life for those needing answers. But mostly, I am thankful that this condition is not debilitating or life-threatening and that I'll be around for my children for a long time."

Nicole

"My story begins in 1975, when, at the age of five, I was diagnosed with MVP. I was told I was the youngest person to ever receive the diagnosis. I retell that story with great fervor as if it were a fishing legend. I have always known about my heart. I recently read about so many others who obtain a diagnosis only after visiting countless practitioners and having their list of symptoms fall on deaf ears. Although I should probably consider myself lucky to have grown up knowing my diagnosis, I don't. It is difficult to be different in any way at all; having MVP is no exception. As a young child I was required to see a cardiac specialist at UCLA in Southern California every year until I was 15. My memories of these experiences are less than favorable. My poor parents would have to spring the trip on me the morning of the appointment by bribing me with gifts and hoping for the best. I was always told that my heart was just like a squeaky door that made noise but open and shut, doing its job reliably and without question. They said, 'A person without MVP will live to be 100 and a person with MVP will live to be 101.' My concern was, if there was never ever anything to worry about, why all the testing and monitoring? No doctor has ever answered that question to my satisfaction.

> My concern was, if there was never ever anything to worry about, why all the testing and monitoring? No doctor has ever answered that question to my satisfaction.

"I worry. I have been afraid of things my entire life. My earliest memory is of a night terror I had at the age of three. I suffer from panic attacks, obsessive compulsive disorder, generalized anxiety disorder and agoraphobia. I currently take Zoloft and am in a sort of remission. Every time my heart throws extra beats, I am convinced I am dying. Even after suffering bouts of bigeminy that have lasted as long as 60 minutes I am still quite sure that I'll drop dead any minute. All of this nonsense from a tiny, leaky valve."

Carolyn

"Although it is difficult to follow these diet restrictions, I do feel so much better.

"As someone who has been living with MVPS, I want to share the changes I made in my diet and everyday life that have given me great relief from my symptoms. Although it is difficult to follow these diet restrictions, I do feel so much better. First and foremost, avoid all forms of caffeine—both foods and medicines. Carefully read labels. My severe symptoms are triggered by caffeine. Second, daily exercise even if you believe you have no energy. Force yourself—you will feel better. I prefer to exercise early in the morning; it gives me energy for the day. I usually walk briskly, or ride a bike for about 20 to 30 minutes every day. A few times a week, I enjoy a more intense workout. Exercise definitively helps. I learned this the hard way. When I was bedridden for weeks, all of my MVPS symptom returned. When I was able to start exercising, I became symptom-free.

> **Although it is difficult to follow these diet restrictions, I do feel so much better.**

"Third, cut out as much sugar from your diet as possible. This includes high-glucose fruits and juices. Read food labels. If you want something sweet, choose blueberries, strawberries or even wheat crackers. Before bed, I have protein with my sweets right before bed. This helps to stabilize my blood sugar, and thus I avoid feeling sleepy and irritable. My sugar cravings are also less. If I have something really sweet or lots of sweets, I know I am not going to feel well for a few days. To overcome this, I increase my exercise. When I first gave up sugar, it took about two weeks to get it all out of my system. After that, I lost my cravings. Also, avoid artificial sweeteners. For me these triggered my symptoms.

"In essence, eat a well-balanced diet. Consider eating smaller portions more often, as opposed to huge meals. Do this, and you too will feel better."

June

"I am a 53 year-old-woman who has been married for almost 26 years. I have always been a 'Type A' personality—finishing college as an adult in my late 30's and finally getting what I had always wanted—a teaching certificate. I threw myself into my teaching the fall after I graduated from college and the next year began my master's degree. This wasn't merely an education degree. I am a professional classical musician. I had to do several regular performances in order to receive my degrees. Sometime during this college endeavor I began to have minor panic attacks. I just lived with them, figuring that running away from them would do me no good. Sometimes the panic attacks would come right in the middle of playing a huge Bach organ piece or standing up in the choral shell performing some major concert. I managed, however, to live through it all.

"At the same time, late in my bachelor studies, my dad got ALS (amyotrophic lateral sclerosis or Lou Gehrig's disease). My mom and I were the main care-givers. Stress in my life was at an all-time high. I began to have feelings of depersonalization. Actually I noticed these feelings when I was a little tiny kid. The first one I noticed was when I was sitting in church one Sunday. It was the most frightening thing. I told no one, and they continued to happen all through my childhood, but they got much worse during this particular time while in college with my sick dad. I chose to see a free psychologist in the university to discuss my problems because it was getting to be too much. He told me not to worry about the 'phase out' times because they were common during stress. However, it was really scary to be in the middle of an organ recital and suddenly 'coming back' in the middle of it from somewhere—I don't know where my mind actually wandered—but it felt like I wasn't there. I was surprised to see that I was still playing and no one seemed to notice anything.

"All my life I have felt like I was kind of on the outside of things—as if I weren't really totally *in* life. Sort of like phasing in and out at times. I can't really explain, but here's an example. I would walk into a class in high school and everyone would be discussing the test we were going to take. I hadn't ever even heard mention of a test. What test? A test was going to be given that day? That sort of thing happened to me regularly throughout my school days as a kid and teen. I sometimes wonder if my brain gets enough oxygen, although I graduated *magna cum laude* from college and have always gotten excellent grades, read voraciously and try to learn as much as possible. I also usually have a pretty quick wit and have always been able to 'think on my feet,' but I also have these 'phase outs' or feelings of depersonalization. I have always considered myself just a 'music flake'—but actually I think a lot of this is attributable to MVPS.

"In 2002, I had a severe pancreatitis with a gallbladder attack and ended up having my gallbladder removed. Postoperatively I had respiratory problems which prolonged my recovery. In the winter of 2004, I became involved in cross-country skiing. I would be out in the woods, alone sometimes, skiing. I would feel these horrible heart palpitations, similar to previously only not as severe. A 24-Holter (EKG) monitor for 24 hours showed lots of extra beats. This led me to a cardiologist who, after ordering an echocardiogram, diagnosed me with MVP. He prescribed Pindolol, which is a beta blocker. The medication gave me hives. Then he prescribed Toprol XL®. Within a week I became so exhausted I could hardly move. I was sleeping all the time. The palpitations continued with a vengeance. The Toprol wasn't touching them, and the general malaise from the beta blocker kept getting worse. I gained weight. I couldn't exercise because I was just way too exhausted all the time. I bought a blood pressure monitor and discovered that my blood pressure was extremely low. The medication was stopped. I was told that I would have to live with the palpitations.

| Basically, I refuse to give up my enjoyment of life with this silly health problem. |

"The palpitations, however, are a terrible problem. With each episode, I feel a surge of adrenaline which wipes me out for two days. I feel like I'm recovering from the flu. I have to rest in bed; moving is an effort. When stress increases, I can't control the palpitations. What I try to do is get rest, stay hydrated, stay on an exercise program, eat very little sugar, lots of vegetables and healthy food, and control my stress.

"Interestingly my symptoms got worse while I took HRT (hormone replacement therapy) during menopause. Once the strength of the hormones was reduced, my palpitations were less severe.

"MVP isn't my only problem. I'm also being treated for asthma, allergies, gastric reflux, irritable bowel syndrome, chronic sinusitis and arthritic problems. Too I have a curvature in the upper part of my spine, a concave breastbone, extremely long limbs and am very hyperflexible."

"I am thoroughly convinced that there is more to MVP, perhaps some sort of autonomic nervous system disorder. When I cautiously approach this subject with my physician, whom I have known for many years, I merely see a glazed face. He doesn't want to discuss this. Although I have always loved this doctor, I have turned to an alternative sort of treatment. I am currently also seeing a kinesiologist/chiropractor who has been giving me dietary supplements, which seem to help in certain areas such as joint problems and reflux.

"I am very lucky to have an extremely supportive husband. My biggest fear, however, is that I will fall over dead unexpectedly, as my uncle (my mother's brother) did. He had MVP and was out mowing his lawn and just fell over dead. The cardiologist assured me that this is not a possibility, but I don't believe him. I don't know how anyone can know that this will not happen, when they don't even seem to know that MVP is more than just a birth defect. I have basically, however, decided that if that happens then it happens, and I'm not going to stop jogging on the treadmill at the gym or working out with weights because it makes me feel so much better to do those things. Basically, I refuse to give up my enjoyment of life with this silly health problem. I try to see humor in things that used to upset me, or I try to avoid upsetting situations. It's all I can do."

Mike

"I am now 43 years old. When I was 19 and in my sophomore year of college, I began to experience the first symptoms of MVP. I remember times when I would be sitting on the couch watching television and all of the sudden my heart would start beating hard. It was as if I was running and suddenly stopped. At first these episodes were short and infrequent. Soon they became more intense. As days turned into weeks I dropped down to about 90 pounds. I'm 6'1"—which made me *very* skinny. I couldn't sleep at night. I couldn't stay awake during the day. My chest would become tight. My left arm and sometimes even my right arm would ache. I made an appointment with my physician and explained my symptoms. However, at this time my symptoms were episodic. The doctor listened to my heart and told me everything sounded normal to him. He also told me that I should consider myself fortunate to be so thin. Most of his patients were overweight and would like to be thin like me. I decided that this physician was not going to help me, and so I made an appointment with a cardiologist. Strangely enough, the cardiologist told me the same thing, but he did say that I was too young to have heart trouble.

"One night I had been awake almost all night with a pounding heart. I hurt so badly that I thought I was going to die. I asked a friend to drive me to the emergency room. As soon as we got there, my symptoms subsided. Everyone thought I was a nut. Weeks turned into months and school let out for the summer. When I came home for the summer I told my parents that I thought I was having heart trouble. My mother was concerned and made an appointment for me with our family physician. When I went to see him, I was having an episode. The doctor was confounded. He said he didn't know what the problem was, but that I had a serious problem and he was referring me to a cardiologist. When I went to see the cardiologist, they did a number of tests on me. The cardiologist told me that I had a mitral valve prolapse. He did not think it was serious, but if it would make me feel better I could try taking a new experimental drug called Inderal (now a very old beta blocker) that was supposed to help these types of symptoms. I started taking one 10-mg pill four times a day. But the medicine did absolutely nothing for me. A few days later I started having a major episode. I decided that if these pills didn't help me I would surely die, so, instead of taking one pill I took four. After taking four I started feeling a little better. So I took four more. That almost got it, so I took two more for a total of ten pills. Eureka! the Inderal stopped the episode. I started taking between 16 and 20 of these pills a day. As my supply started running out, I knew that the doctor who gave me the prescription would not give me the amount of medicine that I needed, so I made an appointment with another cardiologist and told him I was taking 40 mg four times a day. As time went by I started walking again; because I was so sick I had not been able to exercise, and I knew this would be good for my heart. It was several weeks before I could even walk a mile. But with the Inderal, I was able to not only walk that mile, but to run it and two more six months later. I also began gaining weight back, although I am and have always been thin.

> One night I had been awake almost all night with a pounding heart. I hurt so badly that I thought I was going to die.

"Over the years with the help of the Inderal I have gone on to live a normal life. I am married and have three children. I am a Cub Scout den leader and I teach Sunday school. I took 160 mg of Inderal for several years. Instead of taking it four times a day I started taking 80 mg at lunch and 80 mg before bed. Later I was able to just take 80 mg at lunch and 40 mg before bed. I took Inderal for 20 years. I now take one 50-mg Toprol® at lunch time and am doing quite well."

Lyn

"I was diagnosed in the mid-80s, many years ago, with MVP during a routine check up. I really didn't pay any attention to the diagnosis. When I told my dentist, however, he said I needed antibiotics prior to certain procedures. During the ensuing years, I never heard any physician mention MVP. Then in early 1990 I went to a new internist, who said I did not have MVP. That puzzled me. I believed I did, so I went to a cardiologist who told me I *did* have MVP. I wanted to know because my father also had 'soldier's heart' and my brother had been treated at a major clinic for atrial fibrillation for the last 40 years—he also has MVP.

> I feel like my body is racing inside.

"I don't believe MVP bothers me, but I do wonder whether it's related to my other problems. I had very bad migraines several times a week for about 25 years, but no one has ever said they were related to MVP. My cardiologist prescribed atenolol (a beta blocker), which relieved my migraines. I finally was able to wean myself off the medication and am migraine-free. My worst problem is that I clench my teeth during sleep. This leaves me fatigued and with a headache that's not a migraine. I also feel like my body is racing inside. This happens more so after I take medicine like Sudafed®. Perhaps I have too much adrenaline on board. I try to keep myself informed—that's the only way I can help myself to live with MVP."

Debbie

"I was diagnosed with MVP at age 30—I'm now 41. I still remember that day at the laundromat when my heart suddenly started rapidly pounding, so much so that I thought my heart would bounce out of my chest. After more episodes and a trip to the emergency room, I saw a cardiologist. He prescribed Tenormin® (a beta blocker) and told me to take antibiotics prior to dental visits. The Tenormin slowed my heart to ~50 beats per minute. I became scared and stopped the medicine. Since, I occasional get rapid heartbeats.

"MVP has affected my life. Years ago I was fearless. I traveled, skied, eat everywhere, and rode horses. Then I turned 25 years of age, and became neurotic. I didn't want to travel far from

> I spend lots of energy making excuses to avoid activities with my friends. I don't want to explain my fears.

home, I didn't want to eat in public—what if I choked, and I didn't want to exercise—what if I had a heart attack? Today, I continue with these problems. At the movie theater I sit at the end of the row. What if I have to run out? I'm afraid to walk briskly—my heart might start pounding. In fact, I purchased a bicycle. I thought this was a great idea to get in shape. After riding for a mile, however, my heart started pounding. It took me hours to calm down.

"I'm not presently on any medications. I occasionally experience palpitations—the fluttery kind. They still scare me, particularly when I'm in the midst of teaching. To avoid fainting, I concentrate on my teaching lessons. Thus far I have been very successful. One trick that I discovered that helps me avoid fainting is to bear down by tensing my stomach muscles and pushing. Along with the palpitations are dizzy spells. I keep on teaching and eventually they stop. All the while I can't help thinking, please stop, please stop, please don't let me pass out in front of these children.

"I do feel lucky because I have great friends, a supportive family, a great career and a beautiful home. I'm still single. What's the point of looking for someone? I won't fly, I won't hike, bike or ski and won't go anywhere where I will get to hot. I worry about getting sick. Who would want to be associated with me?

"I continue to live my limited life. I take baby steps on a straight and narrow path. I wish I could do more and not worry as much. Boy does that take lots of energy. I spend lots of energy making excuses to avoid activities with my friends. I don't want to explain my fears. The bottom line is that I'm here and each day, strive to do a little more. Eventually, I will get there."

Candace

"In 1989 I went to an internist with complaints of dizziness, headaches, feeling faint, and surges of adrenal that scared me to death. Through the years, I've been X-rayed, CT-scanned, monitored, echoed, and drained of many tubes of blood. I've had ENT, neurology and ophthalmology work-ups, and after developing extra beats, ended up in the emergency room. Nine years and seven physicians later, it was my daughter, an interior designer, who found MVP syndrome on the Internet. I was so relieved with a diagnosis that I actually cried. Finally I was diagnosed. I'm trying my best not to waste energy on anger. Why don't physicians know about this syndrome? I'm currently suffering from a myriad of symptoms, but as I learn more and network with others, I'm taking more control. I believe I have finally found an internist and a cardiologist that will help me. I keep hoping."

Kathy

"I remember getting palpitations shortly after the birth of my second child. They were sporadic and not very bothersome. I ignored them. A few months later, I began to have chest pains. Relief only came from pressing on my chest with a finger over the painful area. These pains were intermittent. During a routine exam, I mentioned them to my physician who sent me for a chest X-ray. The X-ray was normal. He said I had costochondritis, an inflammation of the ribs.

"Several years passed. I learned to live with the pain and fluttering heart. I lived in Las Vegas, Nevada, and was a stay-at-home mom. I knew I was under a lot of stress but never felt it was a problem. Looking back, I see that I had several symptoms of depression but, at the time, I didn't recognize them. My life changed in February 2001.

"I decided to have porcelain veneers put on my teeth and went to my dentist's office for the first part of the procedure. About an hour after I came home my arms and legs felt heavy and I could barely stand. A searing wave of nausea exploded in my stomach. I collapsed on my bed and thought I must have 24-hour flu. As the hours passed, I started feeling more and more anxious. Suddenly, I could no longer lie down. I got up and paced throughout the house, walking in circles over and over again. I was physically exhausted but my body would not let me stop. If I tried to sit, my leg would move up and down. My mind was reeling

> The epinephrine I received at the dentist's office was enough to trigger the disorder.

"My husband took me to the emergency room, where a series of tests were performed. The doctors found nothing wrong with me and said it must be the flu. Over the next week, I had lost 10 pounds and could not eat a bite of food. I had not slept one minute. I called my dentist who said I must be having some type of an anxiety attack. She put me on Xanax. It didn't help—my anxiety mounted. I knew I was dying. I called my doctors for help and no one knew what to do. I was out of my mind with fear.

"It was time for me to return to the dentist to finish the veneers. Again, after I came home the reaction was so severe. I didn't know how I could make it through another day. My mother lives in San Diego, California and I went to the Scripps Clinic for help. I saw an allergist who thought I must be having some kind of reaction to the Novocain or epinephrine used in the procedure. She determined the epinephrine had likely caused the reaction.

"But why? That was the million-dollar question. I went back home and struggled to get better. My arms and legs were tingling and I had bouts of irritable bowel syndrome, I had a nonstop pounding headache so painful it made my cry. My heart was out of control, wildly beating. At times, I would lose my voice or feel like something was in my throat when there was nothing there. The list can go on and on. I felt like I had no control over my body and everyday some new weird symptom would emerge.

"During this time I saw several doctors who tested me for everything under the sun. All the tests came back negative. A cardiologist, however, diagnosed my having a 'slight' mitral valve prolapse. The doctors were stumped. I just knew they were tired of my complaints. After three months of confusion, I went to a large metropolitan medical center. There I saw an endocrinologist for a presumed thyroid disorder. The doctor took one look at my voluminous medical records and told me this was clearly a case of depression. He put me on an antidepressant and I slowly began to recover. Eventually, I found a psychiatrist in Las Vegas who took over my treatment. Now, four years later, I am fully recovered. With the help of the psychiatrist, the pieces of the puzzle fit. He believes I was genetically predisposed to panic disorder and depression. The epinephrine I received at the dentist's office was enough to trigger the disorder. Too, the symptoms of mitral valve prolapse syndrome can be similar to panic disorder."

Cathy

"Living with MVPS has not been easy for me or for those around me, but I learned how to control it and how to live a normal life.

"As I grew up, I complained about my heart doing flip-flops, speeding up, and then slowing down for no apparent reason. Since no one worried about this, I didn't either. I never imagined what was to follow. I will never forget the night I woke up suddenly with terrible chest pains, shortness of breath, and an unnerving fear that I was dying. 'I'm only 25 years old,' I thought. 'How could I be having a heart attack?'

> I'm only 25 years old. How could I be having a heart attack?

"I refused to go back to sleep—afraid I would never awaken. This was the start of endless symptoms: chest pains, headaches, heart palpitations, panic attacks, shortness of breath, fatigue, dizziness, and even fainting.

"I went to a physician who diagnosed MVP. He, however, ran additional tests that ruled out problems with similar symptoms. These tests came back negative, and the echocardiogram confirmed his diagnosis. Now I had a name for my symptoms—MVP—and a prescription for a beta-blocker supposed to alleviate my symptoms, or so I thought. Other than, 'Do not worry. There is nothing wrong with you,' I received no further information.

> Other than, "Do not worry," I was given no explanations.

"Things worsened. I experienced symptoms daily that affected me, as well as those around me. Three or four times I went to the emergency room for fainting spells only to be told there was nothing life threatening. One physician said, 'Everything is in your head. You cause your own symptoms.'

"How could this be? I was miserable. Out of fear that something might happen, I avoided grocery stores and restaurants. I needed help. I needed to know more about mitral valve prolapse. About that time a co-worker told me about an advertisement on the radio for a seminar on MVP. Now, my life began to look up. Through seminars, and later on through support group meetings I learned how to deal with my MVPS. I now understand what MVP is and why things happen. I no longer fear that I am going to die.

"The greatest help to me was listening to others with MVP and knowing that I was not alone—we shared the same symptoms and fears. I learned how to control my symptoms without drugs. I ride an exercise bike regularly. I eliminated caffeine from my diet, increased my fluid intake, and use salt freely. In the past six months, I've had no severe symptoms. My life is becoming normal."

Karl—*Kathy's husband's point of view*

"My wife, Kathy, first experienced symptoms associated with MVP only about 10–12 months ago. My early reactions, therefore, are relatively fixed in my mind. In the past several months, I went through a cycle that began with fear, then disbelief, relief, annoyance, and finally understanding, and adaptation. Let me explain.

"Kathy often commented in the past that her heart flip-flopped or sped up for no apparent reason. This never bothered either of us till one night she awakened with a full-blown panic attack: chest pains, shortness of breath—the works. This attack eventually passed. Then, when the symptoms recurred, I sensed that something was seriously wrong, but I tried not to let on. After two or three trips to the emergency room, however, I couldn't hide my feelings.

"After four or five weeks of severe symptoms, Kathy was diagnosed with MVP. When I learned this was not life threatening, my first reaction was disbelief. How could something that created such havoc *not* be life threatening? In fact, we even sought other physicians' opinions.

"Eventually, relief set in. I was convinced things were going to be all right. It was very comforting to have two physicians agree that it was MVP and it could be controlled.

"My next stage—annoyance—is hard for me to discuss. I actually felt annoyed with my wife. After all Kathy had been through, I could not understand why she still felt symptoms, still had panic attacks, and still felt lethargic. I wanted to get on with our lives.

"We began to attend seminars and group sessions with other MVP patients. Now, I better understand what Kathy went through. I also understand how important it is for me to be supportive. Since we made some changes and adapted to living with MVP, we both know it is going to be all right."

Fred—*another husband's point of view*

"Husbands and boyfriends also need to become both educated and empathetic about MVPS. Unfortunately, my wife's symptoms sometimes negatively affect our relationship. For example, we forego wonderful activities together, afraid that she may end up in the emergency room with palpitations or a panic attack. Furthermore, her medications cause fatigue and suppress both her emotions and her enthusiasm. Together, the syndrome and the drugs inhibit her spontaneity. I am devoted to my wife and want to do things as a couple. I feel, however, that life is leaving us behind. We are almost forty, slim, fit, and athletic—but, we act as if we're over the hill. Although I surf, run and work out with friends, I want to be with *her*. If I could convince her that an active life-style wouldn't hurt, it would be great.

"At times I feel she ignores me or pushes me aside. She bonds with other people with MVP for support. I want her to bond with *me*.

"To other spouses I say, "Be informed; be supportive; and be optimistic. Repeatedly tell her, 'You are OK.' Don't put your life on hold."

Deborah

"I am not sure exactly when my symptoms began. During my teen-age years, however, I remember a pounding heart for which I took tranquilizers. I was extremely nervous, anxious, and bothered by a lump in my throat.

"About 10 years ago, at the age of 37, my symptoms surfaced and started to control me. I felt I was having a heart attack and was going to die. I had anxiety, pounding heart, palpitations, chest pains, and a fast heart rate. Many times I experienced a tightening feeling in my chest and became scared. I paced the floor; I stretched; I did anything to get rid of the symptoms.

"During that time, on Christmas Eve in 1983, in our presence my father-in-law had a stroke and was taken to the hospital. That night my heart raced, and I experienced chest pain.

"As a result, I went to see a general practitioner—my first mistake. I tried to share symptoms and relate my family history. He stopped me from telling him anything and examined me. "There is nothing wrong with you; calm down," he said. I tried to believe him, but the symptoms were there: the pounding heart, palpitations, chest pain, pain in my arm and jaw that didn't stop. I knew it wasn't all in my head.

> I knew it wasn't all in my head.

"Next, I called my father-in-law's cardiologist, a knowledgeable, soft spoken man. He said it sounded like MVP. I had an echocardiogram and Holter monitoring done. He said I had MVP, shouldn't worry, and that I wasn't going to die. Then, he started me on Inderal. I have been on medication since, and take Ativan when I need it. Over the years whenever my symptoms worsened, he increased my medications.

"I believe MVP controls my life at times. I try not to let it bother me, but sometimes it does. I am grateful for the influx of information on the subject and believe education is the key. How well I remember when I first went on medication. My sister-in-law said, 'Why are *you* under stress? *You* don't work.' I'll never forget it. Just because I wasn't working full time, I shouldn't have stress.

"I don't think my husband understands the impact MVP has had on me. I tried to explain it, but to a person who has never experienced it, I think it is hard to understand. Also, I have never been hospitalized for this or gone to the emergency room. He has never witnessed my having a problem so severe that I am hospitalized.

"What I have read, and now that MVPS is being recognized has helped. Although I still have my moments, it certainly is not like the beginning.

"My 23-year old son has been diagnosed with MVP. He has chest pain occasionally, but he's never been on medication."

Diana

"I am now 60. Until a year ago when I discovered the MVP program, I battled the unknown and survived the trauma of many misdiagnoses. I lived with severe panic attacks, sought professional help, and endured all the bizarre symptoms mentioned in *Taking Control*.

"Twenty years ago, after my husband's death, my life changed. Fear was my constant companion. I white-knuckled my way through graduate school and into a new career. Family, friends and physicians thought I imagined symptoms. As a result, I found myself in isolation.

"After a self-diagnosis of anxiety, I used relaxation techniques, meditation, and drank calming herbs and teas. This lessened my symptoms.

"I enrolled in college—a challenge. I experienced dizziness, fatigue, shortness of breath, and was plagued with chronic shoulder pain. The desire to be thinner meant crash diets. Rather than meals, I drank tea or coffee. My full class schedule and new diet equaled trouble.

"Following college, during the first year of marriage, I worked 14 hours a day, and continued dieting. My symptoms became unbearable. Cardiologists at my husband's medical school diagnosed a heart murmur. They said to curtail all activity. The future looked bleak.

"My mother, not satisfied with the diagnosis, insisted I go to my hometown hospital. After a 24-hour monitor and an echocardiogram, I was diagnosed with MVP. I received information about penicillin use for dental procedures and surgery, and was instructed to resume my normal activities.

"The symptoms continued. At the request of physician friends, I continued to undergo testing. Diagnoses included: hypoglycemia, asthma, hiatal hernia and more. I took medications and suffered side effects. No one connected the symptoms with MVP.

> ... I am now 60 ... I battled the unknown and survived the trauma of every misdiagnosis ...

"Now, with the help of the book and newsletters, I learned to take control. I noticed a tremendous difference when I followed the guidelines for diet, water intake, salt, caffeine, and chocolate. I read letters from others with MVP and feel reassured. I find the 'top ten list' helpful in reducing my anxiety—I refer to it several times a week. My symptoms along with my stress are alleviated by drinking calming herbs. My favorites contain valerian, passiflora, celery seed, catnip, hops, and orange peel."

Dora

"In the summer of 1990, I experienced dizzy spells and feelings of lightheadedness once or twice a week for brief moments. I blamed the summer heat and didn't believe the spells were serious. The dizzy spells lasted three to four weeks. Once they were gone, I didn't give them a second thought. In late November of 1990, the lightheadedness returned, and I experienced nervousness. My hands shook and my legs felt like lead. Because I didn't feel stressed I couldn't understand why I experienced unusual symptoms. I also experienced severe nasal congestion and stuffiness. I thought I was getting the flu or a bad cold.

"Nonprescription decongestants did nothing and made me feel worse. By early December, the symptoms increased in intensity and in frequency. The dizziness progressed. Whenever I walked or stood up from a sitting position, I felt as if I were riding on a fast elevator. I had extreme pain deep inside the middle area of my sinuses. I experienced rapid heartbeat, chest pains, and shortness of breath. I figured this bad case of the flu was out of hand and went to the emergency room. The attending physician could not explain the rapid heartbeat and diagnosed me with sinusitis. He prescribed an antihistamine and decongestant that gave me no relief.

"On the third day after drinking a half cup of coffee with my medication, my heart rate suddenly increased, and I couldn't breathe. I knew I was having a heart attack! Paramedics took me to the emergency room. The EKG, chest X-ray, and blood work were normal. The physician said, 'The flu is in your head. Go home. Don't drink any liquids or take medication with stimulants.'

"A week later, a family practice physician at my HMO also diagnosed me with sinusitis and prescribed mild medication. Nothing alleviated the dizziness, chest pains, or rapid heartbeats.

"Next, I was referred to an ear, nose, and throat specialist. He conducted various tests and said, 'You don't have sinusitis. It's possible you have mitral valve prolapse.' Three weeks passed. Then, an echocardiogram showed I did have MVP. No one explained this condition, and I was not able to speak with a cardiologist. The technicians told me that dizziness is not associated with MVP.

"I persisted with the validity of my symptoms and a CAT scan and Holter monitor were ordered. This physician said the dizziness was due to stress in my life. The CAT scan results were normal. The Holter monitor revealed a fast heartbeat. My physician prescribed Inderal for the rapid beats and Antivert for the dizziness. Although the Inderal helped the rapid heartbeat and chest pains, it made me very tired. I could barely function. It also affected my breathing. The Antivert helped the dizziness.

"Again, I switched physicians and HMOs. I went through the entire process of seeing other family practice physicians, as well as another ENT specialist. I also saw two neurologists, who referred me back to ENT. No one was able to help me. All the physicians I saw seemed baffled by my mysterious symptoms.

> ... I have MVP.
> However, no one
> explained what this is.

"Finally, in November of 1991, I was taken off the Inderal by another family-practice physician, who prescribed Tenormin. By this time the dizziness subsided and I went off the Antivert. From December, 1990 till May, 1991, I was completely incapacitated and out of work—a great financial burden. Talk about stress.

"It was only recently I found information on MVPS. If only I had this years ago. I continue to take a small dose of Tenormin, and it seems to help a little. I eat a healthy diet and do aerobic exercise with strength training three to four times per week. I stopped drinking coffee and soft drinks and limited my intake of desserts. I consume a sports drink that contains natural glucose, no added sugar, and all the major electrolytes. This drink helps. My symptoms lessened. I still experience extra beats and chest pain; however, now I know *why* these symptoms occur and that I *can* do something about them."

Madonna

"In February of 1992, after my second miscarriage, I experienced rapid heartbeats. I saw a physician, who, after an echocardiogram and an EKG, diagnosed mitral valve prolapse. I began with a low dosage of Tenormin, which helped some. It did not, however, help the irregular, rapid heartbeats. I avoided caffeine and alcohol and cut down on sugar, but I felt only minimal relief.

"About a month later, I experienced extreme dizziness and lightheadedness and was treated for fluid in my ears. I was on Antivert for about one month. Shortly after, I stopped taking the Tenormin because I wanted to get pregnant again. Several tests failed to explain my two miscarriages.

"In July of 1992, I miscarried a third time. The pounding heartbeat and dizziness continued, although I found some relief with routine aerobic exercise. After several infertility tests, I had surgery in October 1992 to correct a uterine defect.

"After surgery, I continued to experience extreme dizziness, an irregular-pounding heartbeat, and a constant feeling of being off balance—like being on a boat.

"During the onset of menses when I feel stressed and tired, my symptoms magnify. I have occasional panic attacks, and I feel depressed. To always feel miserable affects both my home life and my job performance. My husband, although very understanding, often feels helpless. I am afraid to go shopping because I get dizzy and panic. I hate how it affects my life, and I hope it goes away as suddenly as it began.

"I was relieved to read *Taking Control: Living with MVPS*, and to learn how other people deal with these symptoms. It helped to know panic attacks can be controlled, that positive steps can be taken. I do feel some relief from symptoms when I maintain a regular exercise schedule. Now, I am concerned about how I will be able to control my symptoms once I get pregnant, since my past history prohibits exercise."

Janet

"I am 27 years old, married and have two beautiful children. When I was five years old my pediatrician detected a heart murmur. It was not serious, and I outgrew it by the age of nine.

"Until the age of 23, my life went quite well. Then, one day when my husband and I were on our way home from Florida, I began to feel funny, tired, and dizzy. I didn't think much of it until a month later when, along with chest pains, my heart raced and palpitated. My husband rushed me to an emergency room. On the way there, I kept telling him I was scared, and I felt as if I were going to die. The physician sent me home and said there was nothing wrong with me.

"Over the next several months, my symptoms became worse. I went to several emergency rooms, and got the same response each time: 'There is nothing wrong with you—it's your nerves.'

"I experienced several anxiety, panic attacks whenever I went out. My heart raced and I felt dizzy—I had to leave. The anxiety was so intense I was scared to leave the house, and I was afraid to be alone. Eventually, I stopped driving; I stopped going anywhere. I went to several physicians and specialists and asked them to help me. One said, 'It's lupus.' Another said, 'It's multiple sclerosis.' A third said, 'It's an inner-ear problem, and you need surgery.' A fourth said, 'No, you don't need surgery.' My symptoms were very real, but the answers went from one extreme to another.

> Eventually, I stopped driving. I stopped going anywhere.

"After one year, I admitted myself into a psychiatric unit. Now, I had an echocardiogram. The physician told me I have MVP. I was relieved to find the cause of my symptoms, but my battle wasn't over. For the next two years, I searched for more answers to help me overcome all the fears. I saw a few other physicians who told me MVP is no big deal. It's something you have to live with.

"When I saw a newspaper ad for a class on MVP, I attended. There, I learned more about MVP in two hours than I had in two years. I joined this clinic's exercise program. When I began, every day I experienced chest pains, palpitations, migraines, fatigue, dizziness, and anxiety attacks. After six weeks of exercising three times a week and following their advice, I noticed a difference in the way I felt. I had fewer symptoms and began to feel like a new person.

"The key to reducing the symptoms and leading a normal life is to understand MVP and to know *how* to help yourself. I am fortunate to have a loving, supportive family."

Necia

"My problem began at a young age, when the medical community seemed unaware that such a problem could exist in a child. My parents took me from physician to physician to no avail. First, I was diagnosed with anemia, given iron tablets, and told to take some type of liquid in grape juice three times a day. To spare my parents any further worry, I followed this prescription and tried to ignore my symptoms. I had nightmares, chest pain, palpitations and tachycardia, as well as fatigue. If any of these problems were due to a stressor, I was unaware. All I knew was at the onset I was miserable and have remained in a self-guarded state to this day.

"In school sports I was never very active—I was always the referee. I played in the symphony orchestra. As a majorette in the band, never once did I complete the parade route. I dropped out because of fatigue. Although I was an honor student and received many awards in academics and music, I did not go away to college. I was afraid to, but no one knew why.

> I visited emergency rooms throughout the country to no avail.

"I married a few years after my high school graduation, gave birth four years later with no problems, and remain happily married. During those years, however, I experienced numerous problems due to my condition and visited emergency rooms throughout the county to no avail. Never, until recent years, did I go to an emergency room where the staff knew what my symptoms meant. All they knew was I had a rapid, irregular heartbeat that meant trouble.

"Finally, in 1981, I was correctly diagnosed. After a scary emergency room visit and with an extremely rapid pulse that lasted for over an hour, I was admitted to the cardiac care unit and seen by a cardiologist. An angiogram—dye test of the coronary arteries—revealed that my arteries were fine. He diagnosed me with idiopathic supraventricular tachycardia (SVT), and said the cause was unknown. It may come on at any time, may disappear for years, and then surface at a later time. There were no instructions for my follow-up. He gave me Lanoxin and Valium, and told me to resume my life. Because I lived with this for so long with no help, I went home to live with it again.

"After taking Valium for three months and sleeping my life away, I threw the pills away and begged the physician for help. An echocardiogram revealed MVP. So now I had MVP. What a relief, but still there was no help. My primary care physician was sympathetic, but I don't believe he knew what to do.

"During my menses, my condition worsened. I would stay in bed for a week. I decided to seek help because of heavy bleeding, headache, and extreme abdominal pain. I saw a gynecologist who suggested hormone therapy. After an examination, he recommended a hysterectomy. After the hysterectomy I felt better than I had since I was a child. Ten years later I still am thankful to that gynecologist and to my primary care physician for working together to relieve me of that misery.

> I always believed it was all in my head.

"After the surgery, I returned to work full time, but the fatigue still plagued me. For several years, after work all I could do was fix dinner, maybe clean up the kitchen, and drop into bed. Then I started a walking program. Now I came home with more energy. I walked regularly for quite a while.

"Next, our son enlisted in the U.S. Marine Corps. We built a new home on the other side of the county, and I started an even more stressful job in a law office. For the next seven years I did well, except for occasional tachycardia and fatigue. Then in December 1992, while at work, the tachycardia started and I could not get it under control. I went to the emergency room. Within an hour I converted on my own. I was exhausted.

"I made a follow-up appointment with a cardiologist, a wonderful, caring man. He followed my digoxin level for months and increased the dose. He also prescribed Buspar to help my panic attacks—although I did not know these were panic attacks. He instructed me to walk only for 20 minutes every other day and to not exercise any more than that. I followed his advice until late 1993.

"Because that last trip to the emergency room really scared me, I quit my job. After eight months of loneliness, I returned to work. During the time I was at home, I suffered few bouts of tachycardia.

"One day I saw an advertisement for an MVP program, called, and was sent information on a book, *Taking Control*. My prayers were answered. I read it cover to cover repeatedly, and I am grateful it was written. I have lived with this nightmare 43 years with no idea what I could do about this condition. Time and time again physicians said, 'Don't worry; it won't kill you.' I, therefore, believed it was all in my head.

"Now that I have a real handle on things, my palpitations and tachycardia don't bother me much. I no longer feel I'm in a life-threatening situation. The aftermath of exhaustion and irregular heartbeats following the tachycardia, however, take a toll on my health. Instead of hours, it now takes days to recover. I fear that as I grow older these bouts will continue to take a toll.

"I lived this nightmare by myself for 43 years. Now, it is good to know that I am correctly diagnosed, that my condition is not life threatening, and that the medical community recognizes and treats this condition. I follow advice concerning good nutrition and walk again on a regular basis.

"Although I still have hard beats, extra beats, and very short bouts of tachycardia, I feel rather well."

April

"I think my symptoms started when I was nine years old. I would wake up and tell my parents I thought I was dying. My mother would stay up with me till dawn. When it began to get light outside, I felt safe enough to fall asleep. Finally, my parents scheduled a physical. The physician assured them nothing was wrong, but that I was a very emotional child. Through adolescence and into my high school years, I was constantly fearful. My fingers occasionally became numb, and I experienced shortness of breath.

"After age 25, my symptoms intensified. I often awakened from a sound sleep frightened and short of breath. My heart palpitated, my arms ached, and I became numb around my mouth. Although I tried to calm myself and think that it's only stress, I knew better. I continued, however, to cope on my own.

"After years of anxiety and fear, I became totally frustrated. Repeatedly, I awakened at night and asked my husband to take me to the hospital. I knew I was going to die—I was in shock. Time and time again we raced to the hospital only to be sent home. The physician assured us nothing was physically wrong.

I made an appointment with a psychiatrist, who prescribed sleeping pills for the night and nerve pills for the day. I wanted to know what was wrong. I asked her to put me in the hospital, run tests, and give me a complete physical examination—which she did. Still, nothing seemed wrong.

> Time and time again we raced to the hospital only to be sent home.

"Previous symptoms worsened. I was afraid to take the prescribed medicine because I wanted to live a normal life—to not be dependent upon medication. I tried hard to cope on my own. If I awakened, I read, did housework, or paced the floor. No one ever understood how I felt. Everyone suggested that I think more positively. Perhaps I was a hypochondriac! Try as I did, the problems remained.

"I explained to my gynecologist that I experience numbness around my mouth and a heavy feeling in my chest and arms. He admitted me to the hospital and removed a cyst from my ovary. Now that he found something wrong, I felt relieved. Perhaps I'll recover.

"During the first week following my release from the hospital, I could not sleep. For two or three weeks I averaged only two or three hours nightly. I felt as though a heavy rock rested on my chest. My arms ached. I put Bengay on them and a heating pad on my back. Nothing gave me relief.

"Again, I entered the hospital for more tests. My physician finally diagnosed MVP. At first, that scared me to death. I had a heart condition. I read books, and other literature and learned about MVP. The more I studied, the better I understood what went on inside of me for many years.

"As I go to the center to exercise and learn more about MVP, I become less fearful. It is wonderful to be involved with the MVP support group, with people who have had similar experiences. It feels good to have people finally understand me. I feel confident that with continued professional help, I will continue to conquer my fears."

Elizabeth

"As I sat in my high school physics class, I suddenly felt an odd fluttering in my chest. That's when it all started. For the next several months I made several visits to the emergency room for bouts of rapid heart rate. They said it was caffeine. On a second visit, a cardiologist suggested mitral valve prolapse and did an echocardiogram. Through my family physician, he ordered a Holter monitor. Neither physician found a sign of mitral valve prolapse.

"My family physician assured me it was just a minor arrhythmia in my heart—probably caused by stress and not dangerous. He prescribed Inderal. Because I was *not* under considerable stress, I became disturbed. I wanted to know why this happens. In fact, I hoped they really would find a prolapsed valve. Then, I would at least know what I had and that it wasn't serious.

"Fortunately, because I enjoyed dance, my cardiovascular fitness was optimal. Once I began the prescribed medication, I felt fine. Soon afterward I married and moved to Orlando. For peace of mind, I saw a cardiologist. He conducted a Doppler echocardiogram and found MVP. He never mentioned the syndrome, and I had almost no symptoms for three years.

"About six months ago, I experienced more fluttering and occasional arm pain. This started after I had gone a year without regular aerobic exercise. My job became more stressful, and I made some changes. I increased my intake of magnesium, iron, and fluids. I virtually cut out sugar and began aerobics again. I also prayed a lot—What results! I feel much better. A positive attitude helps. This syndrome is frustrating, but remember your body belongs to you—you don't belong to it. Take control."

Terry

"I am a 40-year-old female diagnosed with MVP two years ago. 'MVP is not a big deal,' said my physician. 'Live your life as normal.'

> **Any exertion or any emotional change set off my symptoms.**

"My normal life, however, fell apart two years ago. I suffered with stress, anxiety, and panic attacks. I had more and more days of feeling bad, and I did less and less. Any exertion or any emotional change set off such symptoms as a pounding heart, tired legs, fatigue, and lightheadedness. I lived like a robot. My family fell apart around me. They resented my feeling sick all the time. As symptoms worsened, I became disgusted, frustrated, angry, and depressed. I become agoraphobic—my fears overwhelmed me.

"Then, something happened. A challenge came my way that I really wanted to meet. I knew, however, that the way I felt made it impossible to do so. I realized to feel better, I had to make changes.

"I finally found a physician who understood MVPS. He put me on medication that helped some, but not enough. Next, I attended an MVP seminar and learned so much. I wasn't going crazy; I wasn't losing my mind; and I wasn't going to die. I saw a way out of this vicious cycle that was ruling my life. I could now take charge. Out of shape, and with fears to overcome, I started a regular, low-level exercise program upon which I gradually build. I became more aware of my diet. I limited my intake of sugar and also kept fluid levels up.

"I am in a program to help me deal with agoraphobia. I aim to control my mental attitude and do not fight my symptoms and feelings. I take one day at a time. Although I have bad days, each day I take another step forward to break that vicious cycle. There is much to learn, and I am truly excited."

Arlene

"I first experienced MVP when I was 30 and pregnant with my second child. I drank several cups of coffee before bedtime and couldn't sleep because of palpitations. Thereafter, I avoided caffeine and experienced no more symptoms. Three years later I was hospitalized with an irregular heartbeat for which I took two medications. It was a terrifying experience. Shortly afterward, my physician diagnosed MVP.

> My symptoms included a fluttering feeling in my chest, and most terrifying of all a racing heartbeat.

"That happened nine years ago. I learned to live with my condition, in spite of trying times. My symptoms included headaches, fatigue, palpitations, and dizziness, as well as a fluttering feeling in my chest, and—most terrifying of all—a racing heartbeat. Sometimes I feel as though I walk around in a cloud. I hate all of this.

"I started an aerobic exercise program that enabled me to go off all medication except for a half pill each day. I felt good about that. After three months, due to a couple of episodes of extremely rapid heart rate that lasted two or three minutes each, I went back on the medication.

"I now walk or ride my stationary bike daily and do well. Severe symptoms come and go during flare-ups that last several days. It's upsetting. I can't work outside my home. It's difficult to plan ahead for a nice trip. It sometimes bothers me that my problem makes things harder for my husband and sons.

"Since I receive the newsletter, *Network*, I feel hopeful knowing that many others share my problem. Now, I know there are things—both mental and physical—that we can do to feel better."

Ida

"Eleven years ago as I approached menopause, I first experienced extra heartbeats. A physician, alarmed about my extra beats, sent me to the hospital by ambulance. I was really afraid. After tests, a cardiologist said I have MVP. My doctor told me not to worry—that it was a benign condition. My symptoms became worse—dizziness, headaches, anxiety, together with extra beats, difficult swallowing, sleep problems, ringing in my ears, and shortness of breath. I was started on Inderal and Xanax. After two years on Xanax, I became full of anxiety to the point where I couldn't go into stores. To get off Xanax, I took Ativan.

"I no longer take antidepressants, and my whole life has changed. I feel normal again, although I still have various MVP symptoms. The book *Taking Control* saved my sanity. I am no longer afraid. Recently my physician put me on Tenormin. It didn't help much, so now I am coming off it, too. I want to see whether I can take control by increasing fluids, cutting down on sugar and caffeine, and by walking. So far, this really helped me. I only wish I knew this years ago. I have had problems for ten years."

Linda

"I am a 26-year-old who was finally diagnosed with MVP two and one-half years ago. Being diagnosed was not easy. Some physicians would not listen to my symptoms. I experienced panic attacks, migraine headaches, shaking hands, unusual fatigue and severe mood swings.

"When I could no longer keep it to myself or take another pill, I again sought help. I explained my symptoms to the physician, and that I recently graduated from college, received an offer to teach, and planned to soon marry.

"He said I was under stress and prescribed Buspar. When, after a year, symptoms continued, and I was accused of suffering from PMS 365 days a year, my sister, the nurse, took over. She insisted that I be tested for MVP. My physician reluctantly complied. I had an echocardiogram, and it revealed MVP. I felt relieved because, at times, I thought I was losing my mind. Some days headaches drove me insane, and I felt like jumping out of my skin. Now, the physician prescribed Inderal.

> I was accused of suffering from PMS 365 days a year.

"One recent episode really frightened my husband and me. Throughout the day, I suffered palpitations, lightheadedness, and numbness in the left arm. I returned from a friend's house breathless and felt as if someone were squeezing my heart. Numbness in my left arm continued.

"At the emergency room, I had an EKG. I was told I had a 'prolapse episode.' Again my sister began her research. She told me to call the MVP program for information. This information changed my lifestyle for the better. I cut out caffeinated products such as coffee, tea, and soft drinks. With difficulty, I cut down on chocolate.

"In retrospect, my husband remained a gem. I can't help wondering what might have happened to our marriage if I were continuously misdiagnosed. Although I still have days when I feel exhausted, it helps to be knowledgeable about MVP. I now take control of my life.

"I thank my family, my friends, my co-workers, and especially my mother—who offered prayers. You dealt with me during mood swings; you love *me* for the person I am; and I love *you*. Please wish me luck. My next venture is to get pregnant."

Phyllis

"At age 40 I still experience forceful heartbeats that began fifteen years ago. I especially notice them whenever I relax and lie on the couch.

"Because my mother's early death had been preceded by continuing symptoms of palpitations, lightheadedness, and nausea, I shared my concern with my physician. Although he said I was too young to worry about heart trouble, he ordered an electrocardiogram. Nothing unusual showed up.

"Shortly afterward a friend said she was diagnosed with MVP. Although her symptoms resembled mine, I paid little attention. I come from a family that believes that as long as you can function in your life, don't worry about it. In fact, you have to be half dead before you go to the physician. I felt pretty sure, however, that I did have MVP. Meanwhile, I learned that several years ago four of my sisters had similar symptoms. Two were on medication for palpitations and racing heartbeats.

"Two years ago I suffered from severe stress in the form of TMJ, which my dentist eventually helped me control. A year later, I developed chest pains that recurred during stress. Sometimes, I controlled them by breathing deeply. Unfortunately, the stress and the pains continued.

> I didn't want to do anything, to go anywhere, nor to entertain anyone.

"I withdrew from my family and from my friends. I did not want to do anything, to go anywhere, nor to entertain anyone. All I wanted to do was sleep. Furthermore, I couldn't worry about *my* problems because my little boy began to suffer with medical and scholastic problems. It got to the point where I felt exhausted all the time. My house was a mess. I became irritable, and I rejected my husband.

"After a year I felt half dead, and I became desperate. I visited another physician and explained the forceful heart beat and he said it sounded like MVP. But he told me that my other symptoms are not usual with MVP. After blood work, chest X-ray, EKG, echocardiogram, and an upper GI test, he said my blood count was too low, and confirmed I had MVP.

"For a month I took iron pills to alleviate chest pains and fatigue. The physician believed that because the heart works harder in MVP, that might be the reason for the chest pain. To me, this made sense. After taking iron I felt better. Chest pains became less frequent, less severe. Instead of feeling exhausted by 2:30 P.M., I now remain active till at least 5:30 P.M.

"After my blood count became normal, however, the pains returned. One evening, during a very stressful week, I had a Pepsi. I couldn't get to sleep. The pains were more intense. My friend urged me to call my physician and explain the problem. I hesitated because I felt I bothered him. Although he did not believe my symptoms or physical makeup were typical of angina, he ordered a thallium stress test. The test was normal, and he prescribed Tenormin. After one week I became spaced out and almost passed out. Another time I became confused at the grocery store, unable to make decisions.

> I felt depressed, crazy, and began wondering if it was all in my head.

"My physician cut the medication to half a dose. He suggested that I periodically check my blood pressure since beta blockers sometimes lower it. Although the chest pains were less severe and less frequent, I continued to feel spaced out. Next, he suggested another medication—Inderal.

"Because my husband planned a trip to San Diego and I wanted to feel good, I decided to stop the Tenormin and to not take the Inderal. I still felt tired and spaced out. As my husband and I walked the beach morning and evening, and walked afternoons to sight see, pains became less frequent and less severe. Fatigue remained.

"Upon my return, I again called my physician because I felt pressure on my chest, and I was tired. He said all my tests were normal, and that he didn't tell me I *had* to take Inderal. I felt depressed, crazy, and began thinking it was all in my head. I knew it wasn't. He didn't say I was crazy, but I felt he thought I was a hypochondriac.

"A friend saw something on television about an MVP program and gave me a number to call. I did, and in turn, received valuable information. Now, I knew for sure I wasn't crazy. In fact, I was livid. Had I known about choices other than medication, I would have chosen exercise and diet. It's a shame many professionals don't know more about MVP, don't know how to treat it, and don't know alternatives other than medication.

"I want to tell others to persist. Insist upon more tests until you find out what's wrong. Don't be intimidated as I was and assume you don't know what *you're* taking about."

Vickie

"Approximately six years ago as I stood in the middle of my living room, my heart palpitated for the first time. Prior to that I felt chest pains that lasted only a short time. Then, palpitations began on a regular basis, especially when I was driving. As chest pains came more frequently, I noticed several other symptoms—fatigue, dizziness and pain in both my arms and legs. I sought help from several physicians with no success. Finally, I visited one who gave me a complete physical. He found my electrolytes were low and I showed slight signs of hypoglycemia and low-lying asthma. He sent me to the hospital for testing. A spinal tap showed nothing. A lung test indicated slight asthma, and an echocardiogram showed MVP. He prescribed Tenormin once a day in the morning. I took the medication and my palpitations subsided; however, I felt sick and dragged out.

"About this time I visited a cardiologist who put me on Inderal. I saw him regularly till he moved.

"For a few months afterward I improved. Then, my symptoms worsened. My previous physician told me to go back on Tenormin, and to take it easy. He said not to exercise too much—exercise would worsen my symptoms.

"Tenormin controlled my palpitations, but again I felt sick and dragged out. Again, I switched physicians when my medical insurance coverage changed. My new physician checked and rechecked my symptoms. I explained that my palpitations affected my ability to drive, and she suggested I see a counselor. She kept me on Tenormin and tried a calcium blocker to see if it would help. It did not.

"I met a young lady with MVP who recommended her physician because he controlled her symptoms with medication. Her doctor prescribed Lopressor and Xanax. They helped for awhile. When I tried to stop the Xanax, I felt like a lunatic. Apparently, I experienced withdrawal symptoms. I finally weaned myself and took it when my palpitations seemed they wouldn't stop. Xanax worked within 10 to 15 minutes, but it made me drowsy.

> **When my symptoms are bad, I have a dread fear of impending death.**

"My symptoms ranged from palpitations, anxiety, pain in my neck, numbness in my face, pain in my arms and legs, to tingling in my face and legs. Also, my nerves seemed to be shot. Frequently, whenever I drove my car, I became short of breath and experienced a swelling in the left side of my chest. Then palpitations followed. The palpitations were severe enough that I felt helpless—as if I were dying. Sometimes I wished I would pass out to rid myself of these horrible feelings. The symptoms occurred without any pattern, and would induce an anxiety attack when I was fearful of what might occur.

"When I relax, I sometimes feel anxious, short of breath, and experience palpitations, as well as a swelling in my chest. When the symptoms become intolerable, I am frightened. I make plans with a friend and cancel because I feel bad. Friends sometimes think I'm crazy. They think all I have is a phobia about driving. I saw a psychologist who told me to drive with a friend in the car. Sometimes I feel that I do have a phobia that develops from my fear of symptoms.

"One day I read an article about people with MVP and immediately called for information. I was elated. I joined the program and exercised three times a week at the Center. I stopped my medications and noticed no difference in my symptoms. Six weeks later, I felt a difference. Anxiety and palpitations lessened, and the exercise felt great.

"Four weeks later, however, anxiety and palpitations again started every other day. Once I called 911 when I could not stop the palpitations after an hour and a half. Paramedics said both my pulse and blood pressure were up and my heartbeat was irregular. I refused to go to the emergency room because I had been there several times before to no avail. They tell you to relax. How can you when your heart is beating so rapidly? It's been six months since I discontinued my medication, and my symptoms now appear only 50 percent of the time. Once, I went an entire month without a panic attack.

"I attend an MVP support group and finally learned what causes my anxiety attacks and how to control them. Although I still have some fears and palpitations, I'm learning to deal with them. I realize panic attacks don't come out of the blue. At times I feel some anxiety about what might happen, or what angered me. When I pace myself and stop and relax between tasks, I have minimal anxiety. If, however, I allow myself to be pressured, anxiety from my symptoms turns into full-blown panic attacks. These are horrible—I avoid them at all cost."

Kathryn

"My MVP symptoms started during a trip to China one year after retirement. Steady left-sided chest pains led to one night's stay in the emergency room. At home, two days later, a cardiologist gave me an echocardiogram that confirmed his diagnosis—MVP. 'Live a normal life; ignore the heart pounding; and take walks. Your condition is not life threatening nor serious,' he said. He prescribed beta blockers, but I did not take them.

"Over four months, I gradually regained energy and assumed a semi-normal routine. My family physician advised me to drink more water, to use salt, and to walk. Three months later, after an appendectomy, I felt more tired. My family physician believed adrenalin surges caused my symptoms. He advised me to pace myself. My symptoms worsened. Now, I experienced chest pains, and severe nightly palpitations—severe enough that I was afraid to sleep. Twice within a week I went to the emergency room. The first time, I received a prescription for Valium and Inderal and was sent home. The second time, at my request, I was admitted and saw my cardiologist. He ordered a treadmill test and Holter monitor; both were normal.

"The cardiologist then referred me to a psychiatrist to treat my anxiety. The psychiatrist said, 'Your're running on empty,' and prescribed Xanax.

"Next, my family physician discontinued Inderal and started Tenormin. I took these medications only during potentially, stressful situations. At this time, I heard about and bought the book, *Taking Control*. After reading the book, I finally understand MVP and how to deal with it.

"Instead of Xanax, I later switched to Zoloft, which I continue to take, but in a lesser dose. Like others with MVPS, I experienced periods of not wanting to leave the house. I struggled for enough energy to function on a daily basis. With support from friends and health professionals, I improved. A health therapist convinced me I did not *have* to return to work until I am well, and when I *do* return, it should be for love—not for duty. She referred me to another therapist where, twice a month, I have acupressure and a massage. I joined relaxation classes that follow the Jon Kabat-Zinn program of stress reduction and learned how to relax—something I never knew how to do. I learned deep breathing, body scan, and sitting with awareness. Gradually, I resumed my work, and I continue to remain active. Occasionally, in times of stress, I slow down for a day or two, take a quarter of a Xanax, and—even more rarely—a Tenormin.

"I enjoy hatha yoga. It emphasizes deep, slow, breathing and meditation. Hatha yoga also complements the massage treatments and awareness training. These activities, as well as regular walking, increased my energy and diminished my symptoms. I am grateful for all the treatment, classes, and readings. I have a new understanding."

Bonnie—*a mother's point of view*

"As a mother with MVP syndrome, I find it difficult to deal with the fact my three children inherited this dominant gene. They are now young adults. However, why their lives were such a struggle was apparent only four years ago.

"We spent a great deal of time seeing physicians and enduing many medical tests. The children frequently missed school. Two were even hospitalized—still without a diagnosis. My heart broke when they were told to tough it out and overcome their anxieties on their own. They were made to feel that somehow they were causing their own problems—that they were weak.

"I used to say, 'Why us? Why can't we live like a normal family?' But, today we remain much stronger and much closer than most families because we suffered together.

"I regret that I knew very little about MVPS when my children were growing up. Now, however, I *do* know and I intend to help others."

Toni and George

To conclude, let us share information about *bargaining*, a technique that encourages communication and helps people solve problems.

MVPS affects individuals, as well as those around them— particularly family members. We, therefore, *especially* urge spouses to attend the education seminars. Their responses have been similar: "I'm glad I came." "Now, I understand that my wife [husband] is not the only one and isn't really crazy." "She really *doesn't* make excuses. Often times, she *can't* do something or go somewhere." "The seminar helped us to better understand what she is experiencing."

A true story follows. Toni, a mother of six children between the ages of nine months and ten years, came with her husband George to the Center. Toni was sick and tired of all her symptoms. George was sick and tired of all her complaints. They both needed to find out what's wrong.

Toni was diagnosed with MVPS, and both she and George received much helpful information. A staff member recommended a home-exercise, walking program because of their geographical location and their financial difficulties. Toni became angry. Because of six children, she seldom left the house—even to go for a walk. She seldom enjoyed any free time. No doubt this pressure aggravated her symptoms. Furthermore, both said it was impossible to find anyone to watch all six children.

"Why not let George help?" asked the staff member.

"Oh, no," said Toni. "I never hear the end of it when he has to watch the kids."

A discussion ensued. "She constantly complains," said George. "And, she doesn't want me to go out with my friends in the evening."

Toni thinks George doesn't understand her. George thinks Toni doesn't understand him. Obviously, anger, frustration, and bitterness prevailed. Each one complained about a lack of compassion. Because of their apparent, unsolvable problems, the staff member recommended *bargaining.*

Bargaining, a process, is a type of reciprocal behavior—something for something. For example, a couple bargains for something of equal value—something tangible, something measurable, something with a time limit.

First, each person cited a behavior that is a priority. Said Toni, "I want free time all to myself. Let George watch the kids and not complain." Toni defined free time, and George understood its meaning.

George said, "I want to go out with my friends one evening a week without Toni complaining."

They both agreed to honor their bargains for three months. One month later when asked how their bargaining was going, the response was positive. Furthermore, Toni noted a substantial decrease in her symptoms. They used bargaining with their ten-year-old son. He argues less, and he's more manageable.

As you already know, with MVPS both the symptoms and the individuals' reactions to them often present problems. Symptoms affect persons with MVPS, their families, and their friends. Symptoms may also affect working relations in a negative way. Frequent absenteeism places demands on co-workers.

Remember—there really is a light at the end of the tunnel. Learn all you can about MVPS. Share information with your family and with your friends. With a positive attitude, you will make necessary adjustments in the way you live.

References

Lederer, W. & D. Jackson. 1968. Mirages of Marriage. W.W. Norton & Co. New York.

Padberg, J. 1975. Bargaining. *Perspectives in Psychiatric Care* **13:** 68–72.

Satir, V. 1967. Conjoint Family Therapy, 2nd ed. Science and Behavior Books. Palo Alto, CA.

Sills, G. 1980. Nursing 806.01, Clinical Supervision. The Ohio State University. April.

The Importance of
Proper Food and Fluid Intake

By yourself—and without prescribed medications—you can decrease, and perhaps even abolish your symptoms. How? Data obtained from the MVPS Health Concerns study support previous clinical anecdotal evidence that non-drug interventions work. The table below lists commonly reported measures that lessen symptoms. So carefully study this chapter and then *use* what you learn about the following:

TABLE 4-1. FACTORS THAT LESSEN MVPS SYMPTOMS (*N* = 837)

	N	%
Adequate rest	600	72
Avoiding stress	580	69
Avoiding caffeine	534	64
Regular exercise	511	61
Increased water intake	440	50
Balanced diet	373	45
Other	208	25

This chapter aims to answer the most fundamental questions about how you can steer yourself toward feeling better.

■ **The importance of good nutrition**

Why should I avoid caffeine?
Why should I use salt?
Why should I measure my intake of fluid?
Why concern myself with ill effects of crash diets?
Why and how should I limit my intake of sugar?
Why and how may foods possibly trigger migraines?
Why and how may a magnesium deficiency possible affect me?

■ **The negative effects of some non-prescription drugs**

Do some contain too much caffeine?

Do some stimulate the sympathetic system and worsen my symptoms?

■ **The positive effects of mind over matter—Move it. Exercise. Meditate.**

Why do symptoms cause me to panic, and what can I do?

Can pursed-lip breathing help to overcome shortness of breath?

Which techniques can I use to help relieve chest pains associated with MVPS?

Does stress exacerbate MVPS symptoms, and can I be helped through mindfulness meditation?

■ **The benefits derived from tangible feedback**

Why should I monitor my progress with a *symptom checklist?*

If I study and conscientiously use non-drug intervention, may I be surprised at the end of a 12-week period?

Nutritional Aspects

Why Should I Avoid Caffeine?

Over 80% of the word's population ingests caffeine daily. Most people were first exposed to caffeine *in utero.* That is, many women consume caffeine while pregnant and caffeine readily crosses the placenta. Many children also consume caffeine, at least sporadically, with caffeine use increasing during adolescence and early adulthood, particularly as soda and "energy drinks." Caffeine is rapidly absorbed from the stomach into the bloodstream. Once absorbed, caffeine exerts a variety of physiological effects.

Caffeine stimulates the sympathetic nervous system. Too much caffeine can cause nervousness and jitters. It may also increase your blood pressure (BP). For example, *acute* blood pressure elevations in the range of 5–15 millimeters of mercury (mmHg) are typical following experimental administration of caffeine (2–5 cups per day.) These effects may last several hours. When caffeine is added to emotional stress and cigarette smoking, further increases in blood pressure can be seen. Long-term effects, however, are controversial. Some research found

TABLE 4-2. CAFFEINE CONTENT OF SOFT DRINKS[a]

Company	Brand	Milligrams of Caffeine 8 oz. serving	Milligrams of Caffeine 12 oz. serving
The Coca-Cola Company			
Carbonated Soft Drinks			
	Barq's root beer	15	22
	diet Barq's root beer	0	0
	Barq's Floatz	15	22
	Cherry Coca-Cola	23	34
	diet Cherry Coca-Cola	23	34
	Coca-Cola classic	23	34
	diet Coke	31	45
	diet Coke with lemon	31	45
	diet Coke with lime	31	45
	diet Coke with Splenda	23	34
	Coca-Cola Zero	23	34
	Coca-Cola C2	23	34
	Inca Kola	25	37
	diet Inca Kola	25	37
	Mello Yello	35	51
	diet Mello Yello	35	51
	Mello Yello Cherry	35	51
	Mello Yello Melon	35	51
	diet Mr. Pibb	27	40
	Pibb Zero	27	40
	Pibb Xtra	27	40
	Red Flash	27	40
	TAB	31	47
	Vanilla Coke	23	34
	diet Vanilla Coke	31	45
	Vault	47	70
Teas			
	Nestea lemon sweet	11	16
	Nestea diet lemon	11	16
	Nestea Honey Lemon Green Tea	26	39

TABLE 4-2. (*continued*) CAFFEINE CONTENT OF SOFT DRINKS[a]

Company	Brand	Milligrams of Caffeine 8 oz. serving	Milligrams of Caffeine 12 oz. serving
	Nestea raspberry	11	16
	Nestea sweetened	17	26
	Nestea unsweetened	17	26
	Cool from Nestea	11	16
	diet Cool from Nestea	7	11
	Cool Peach Frrreezer	4	6
	Cool Raspbrrry Cooler	4	6
	Nestea Earl Grey	33	50
Energy Drinks			
	KMX (Orange)	75 per 8.4 oz.	
	Full Throttle	72	
	Sugar Free Full Throttle	72	
Dr Pepper/7 Up			
	A&W Crème Soda	20	29
	diet A&W Crème Soda	15	22
	dn.L	36	54
	Dr Pepper	28	41
	diet Dr Pepper	28	41
	IBC Cherry Cola	16	23
	Ruby Red Squirt	26	39
	diet Ruby Red Squirt	26	39
	Sun Drop Regular	43	63
	diet Sun Drop	47	69
	Sun Drop Cherry	43	64
	Sunkist Orange Soda	28	41
	diet Sunkist Orange Soda	28	41
	Tahitian Treat	Less than 1	Less than 1
Mistic			
	Lemon Tea	12	18
	diet Lemon Tea	12	18
	Peach Tea	12	18

TABLE 4-2. (*continued*) CAFFEINE CONTENT OF SOFT DRINKS[a]

Company	Brand	Milligrams of Caffeine 8 oz. serving	Milligrams of Caffeine 12 oz. serving
Pepsi-Cola Company			
Carbonated Soft Drinks			
	Mountain Dew	37	55
	diet Mountain Dew	37	55
	Code Red Mt. Dew	37	55
	diet Code Red Mountain Dew	36	53
	Pepsi-Cola	25	37
	diet Pepsi-Cola	24	36
	Pepsi Edge	25	38
	Pepsi One	37	55
	Wild Cherry Pepsi	25	38
	diet Wild Cherry Pepsi	24	36
Teas			
	Lipton Brisk, All Varieties	6	9
Energy Drinks			
	AMP Energy Drink (8.4 oz)	75	
Royal Crown			
Colas			
	Royal Crown Cola	28.8	43.2
	Cherry RC Cola	28.8	43.2
	RC Edge	46.8	70.2
Royal Crown Flavors			
	Dr Nehi	28	42
	Kick	38.4	57.6
Nehi Flavors			
	Nehi Wild Red Soda	33.4	50.1

TABLE 4-2. (*continued*) CAFFEINE CONTENT OF SOFT DRINKS[a]

Company	Brand	Milligrams of Caffeine 8 oz. serving	Milligrams of Caffeine 12 oz. serving
Snapple			
	Green Tea with Lemon	16	24
	Ginseng Tea	5	7.5
	Lemon Tea	21	31.5
	Decaffeinated Lemon Tea	3	4.5
	Diet Lemon Tea	21	31.5
	Lemonade Iced Tea	9	13.5
	Lightning (Black Tea)	14	21
	Mint Tea	21	31.5
	Moon (Green Tea)	12	18
	Peach Tea	21	31.5
	Diet Peach Tea	21	31.5
	Raspberry Tea	21	31.5
	Diet Raspberry Tea	21	31.5
	Sun Tea	5	7.5
	Diet Sun Tea	5	7.5
	Sweet Tea	8	12

[a]Source: http://www.ameribev.org/health/caffeinecontent.asp

that people who regularly consume caffeine have a higher average blood pressure than those who avoid caffeine. Conversely, other research reports that regular consumers of caffeine seem to develop a tolerance and, as a result, caffeine doesn't have adverse effects on their blood pressure. To complicate matters, a recent study found that women who consumed caffeinated cola (sugared or low-calorie) had an increased risk of high blood pressure. Researchers speculate that it's not the caffeine, but some other compound found in soda-type drinks that could be responsible for the increased risk of high BP. The data for caffeinated tea are inconclusive.

Caffeine effects on MVPS symptoms, however, are less controversial. It can activate, or worsen many MVPS symptoms. In fact, caffeine can produce anxiety—or panic attacks—in people with panic disorder. Therefore, avoid caffeine altogether.

TABLE 4-3. CAFFEINE CONTENT OF FOODS

Product	Serving Size (oz)	Caffeine (mg)
Coffees		
Coffee, brewed	8	135
General Foods International Coffee, Orange Cappuccino	8	102
Coffee, instant	8	95
General Foods International Coffee, Cafe Vienna	8	90
Maxwell House Cappuccino, Mocha	8	60–65
General Foods International Coffee, Swiss Mocha	8	55
Maxwell House Cappuccino, French Vanilla or Irish Cream	8	45–50
Maxwell House Cappuccino, Amaretto	8	25–30
General Foods International Coffee, Viennese Chocolate Cafe	8	26
Maxwell House Cappuccino, decaffeinated	8	3–6
Coffee, decaffeinated	8	5
Teas		
Celestial Seasonings Iced Lemon Ginseng Tea	16-oz bottle	100
Bigelow Raspberry Royale Tea	8	83
Tea, leaf or bag	8	50
Snapple Iced Tea, all varieties	16-oz bottle	42
Lipton Natural Brew Iced Tea Mix, unsweetened	8	25–45
Lipton Tea	8	35–40
Lipton Iced Tea, assorted varieties	16-oz bottle	18–40
Lipton Natural Brew Iced Tea Mix, sweetened	8	15–35
Nestea Pure Sweetened Iced Tea	16-oz bottle	34
Tea, green	8	30
Arizona Iced Tea, assorted varieties	16-oz bottle	15–30
Lipton Soothing Moments Blackberry Tea	8	25
Nestea Pure Lemon Sweetened Iced Tea	16-oz bottle	22
Tea, instant	8	15
Lipton Natural Brew Iced Tea Mix, diet	8	10–15
Lipton Natural Brew Iced Tea Mix, decaffeinated	8	<5
Celestial Seasonings Herbal Tea, all varieties	8	0
Celestial Seasonings Herbal Iced Tea, bottled	16-oz bottle	0
Lipton Soothing Moments Peppermint Tea	8	0

TABLE 4-3. (*continued*) CAFFEINE CONTENT OF FOODS

Product	Serving Size (oz)	Caffeine (mg)
Caffeinated Waters		
Java Water	.5 liter (16.9 oz)	125
Krank 20	.5 liter (16.9 oz)	100
Aqua Blast	.5 liter (16.9 oz)	90
Water Joe	.5 liter (16.9 oz)	60–70
Aqua Java	.5 liter (16.9 oz)	50–60
Juices		
Juiced	10	60
Frozen Desserts		
Ben & Jerry's No Fat Coffee Fudge Frozen Yogurt	8-oz cup	85
Starbucks Coffee Ice Cream, assorted flavors	8-oz cup	40–60
Häagen-Dazs Coffee Ice Cream	8-oz cup	58
Häagen-Dazs Coffee Frozen Yogurt, fat-free	8-oz cup	40
Häagen-Dazs Coffee Fudge Ice Cream, low-fat	8-oz cup	30
Starbucks Frappuccino Bar	2.5-oz bar	15
Healthy Choice Cappuccino Chocolate Chunk or Cappuccino Mocha Fudge Ice Cream	8-oz cup	8
Yogurts, one container		
Yoplait Cafe Au Lait Yogurt	6	5
Dannon Light Cappuccino Yogurt	8	<1
Stonyfield Farm Cappuccino Yogurt	8	0
Chocolates or Candies		
Hershey's Special Dark Chocolate Bar	1.5-oz bar	31
Perugina Milk Chocolate Bar with Cappuccino Filling	1/3 bar 1.2 oz	24
Hershey Bar (milk chocolate)	1.5-oz bar	10
Coffee Nips (hard candy)	2 pieces	6
Cocoa or Hot Chocolate	8	5

SOURCES: National Coffee Association; National Soft Drink Association; Tea Council of the USA; and information provided by food, beverage, and pharmaceutical companies (J.J. Barone & H.R. Roberts. 1996. Caffeine Consumption. *Food Chemistry and Toxicology* **34**: 119–129).

Although many foods and beverages contain caffeine, it is primarily consumed in coffee. Caffeine content of coffee, tea, cocoa beverages, and foods varies according to the type of coffee bean, tea leaf, or cocoa bean; method and length of brewing; and size of serving. Caffeine content can even vary within the same brand of coffee. For example, it's the highest in drip coffee, and the lowest in instant coffee. Light roasted beans usually have more caffeine than dark roasted coffee beans. (Dark beans are roasted for a longer time, and therefore more caffeine is burned off the bean.) Also, contrary to popular belief, decaffeinated coffee *is not* caffeine-free. Its caffeine content ranges from 2–8 mg per 8-oz cup.

Are you hooked on caffeinated coffee? If so, start weaning yourself now. Mix equal caffeinated and decaffeinated coffee. Use instant coffee—it has the lowest caffeine content. During the next few weeks, continue to add *more* decaffeinated coffee till you are drinking only decaffeinated coffee. If you're addicted to caffeinated tea, follow the same procedure. Don't be alarmed if you experience headaches. Caffeine-dependent people may temporarily suffer headaches for a week or so following withdrawal.

Fluid and Salt Intake

Why Should I Use Salt?

"I have a heart problem. Shouldn't people with heart problems avoid salt?"

Although many MVPers believe this to be true, it is unwise to avoid salt, *unless*, however, you have either *high blood pressure or other medical conditions* whereby salt is restricted.

As explained in Chapter 1, MVPers may have a reduced intravascular blood volume that causes you to become lightheaded and to experience a forceful heart beat upon arising. To increase this volume, therefore, *do not* restrict salt—your source of sodium. In fact, if you aren't using salt, start now. Why?

Approximately 40% of salt is sodium, an essential mineral that retains fluid. Eat salty foods *and* drink water to help increase intravascular blood volume and decrease MVPS symptoms. Although salt comes from natural sources such as meat and fish, most salt comes from processed foods. Examples include soups, pickles, salsa, sauerkraut, and luncheon meats.

Along with maintaining your salt intake, it is very important to drink at least two quarts of water a day. Why? Water is the largest single constituent of the human body. It is essential for cellular homeostasis and life. Studies demonstrate that hydration is especially important for MVPers. The more hydrated a person is, the less are the palpitations, dizziness, lightheadedness and chest pains.

Depending on the amount of lean body mass—the sum of the weight of your bones, muscles, and organs—water accounts for 1/2 to 4/5 of your body weight. In other words, leaner people have a greater percent of body water. Conversely, obese people have a lesser percent body water. On average, men have a higher level of lean body mass than women and therefore have a higher content of body water.

Body water balance depends on the net difference between water gain and water loss. Water gain occurs from consumption of liquids and food, and production of metabolic water produced by oxidation, while water losses occur from respiratory, skin, renal and gastrointestinal tract functions. The National Research Council recommends the following total fluid intake for adults living under average conditions of energy expenditure and environmental exposure: men 3.7 L/day (13 8-oz cups) and women 2.7 L/day (9 8-oz cups).

To be certain to consume enough water, daily pre-measure at least 10 8-oz cups in a pitcher. Subtract the amount that you get on a regular basis for other sources. For example, if you have eight ounces of juice every morning, measure one less cup of water to your pitcher. Keep this pitcher on a kitchen counter, in the refrigerator, or on your desk at work, and take frequent drinks. For convenience, simply carry a 1L bottle of water with you and refill throughout the day. For variety, add an artificially sweetened beverage, herbal tea, or a slice of fresh lemon or lime. Fill the pitcher *daily*, and you'll know exactly how much fluid you regularly consume. Also remember to consume plenty of fruits and vegetables. Although MVPers are wise to avoid caffeinated and alcoholic beverages, data regarding the diuretic effects of caffeine remain controversial. Recent analysis found that doses of caffeine above 250 mg have an acute diuretic effect, whereas single caffeine doses found in commonly consumed beverages have little or no diuretic action. Alcohol, however, has a known diuretic effect, particularly within the first few hours after ingestion.

Do certain factors increase the need for water? Yes. For example, consider the atmosphere in a plane. It may have a very drying effect. Always drink plenty of fluids prior to and during the flight. Be sure to ask for tomato juice—a liquid high in sodium. Too, during any illness accompanied by a fever, your body needs more water. With a fever of 103°, for example, consume at least two or three additional glasses of water daily. High-temperature environments, high altitude, low humidity, and high-fiber diets all increase water requirements. (Specific fluid requirements for exercise are discussed in Chapter 6.)

Finally, avoid using diuretics or water pills. As an MVPer, you may be sensitive to these medications. On the other hand, *if* you take a prescribed diuretic, *don't stop the medication.* First consult with your health-care provider.

TABLE 4-4. WATER CONTENT OF SELECTED FOODS

Food	Water (%wt)	Food	Water (%wt)
Apple, raw	86	Ham, cooked	70
Apricot, raw	86	Lettuce, iceberg	96
Banana, raw	75	Macaroni/spaghetti, cooked	66
Bread, white	36	Milk, 2%	89
Bread,whole-wheat	38	Orange, raw	87
Broccoli,cooked	89	Peach, raw	89
Cantaloupe, raw	90	Peanuts, dry roasted	2
Carrots, raw	88	Pear, raw	84
Cheese, cheddar	37	Pickle	92
Cheese, cottage	79	Pineapple, raw	86
Chicken, roasted	64	Potato, baked	75
Chocolate chip cookies	4	Squash, cooked	94
Corn, cooked	70	Steak, tenderloin, cooked	50
Corn flakes cereal	3	Sweet potato, boiled	80
Crackers, saltines	4	Turkey, roasted	62
Grapes, raw	81	Walnuts	4

SOURCE: USDA National Nutrient Database for Standard Reference, Release 18. Available at: http://www.nal.usda.gov/fnic/foodcomp/Data/SR18/nutrlist/sr18a255.pdf

Postural Orthostatic Tachycardia Syndrome (POTS)

In addition to increasing fluid and sodium intake, further measures may be of help to alleviate symptoms associated with POTS. The first step is to recognize and remove offending agents such as diuretics, antihypertensives (primarily sympathetic blockers), nitrates, and certain antidepressants. Do so with the knowledge of your health-care provider. Do not stop medications unless instructed. Next is to be cognizant of the number of orthostatic demands that occur throughout the day and practical countermeasures. These include:

- Arise slowly, in stages, from supine to seated to standing. This measure is particularly important when first arising in the morning.
- Avoid straining, coughing and walking in hot weather; these activities reduce the amount of blood returning to right side of the heart (venous return) and worsen orthostatic hypotension.
- Sleep with the head of the bed elevated 10 to 20 degrees.
- Wear custom-fitted waist-high elastic stockings. These help minimize pooling of blood in your legs and facilitate blood return to the heart.
- Get regular cardiovascular exercise (discussed in detail in Chapter 6).
- While standing in line, tense your legs by crossing them. This maneuver can increase the amount of blood pumped by your heart.
- Practice getting up from a sitting position.
- While standing, squeeze a small soft material ball with your hand.
- Minimize alcohol intake.
- Avoid eating large meals; eat frequent, small, lower carbohydrate meals.
- Avoid activities or sudden standing immediately after eating.

Crash or Fad Diets

Why Concern Myself with Ill Effects of a Crash Diet?

Because Americans spend millions in search of ways to lose weight, they often become vulnerable to false and sometimes adverse effects of quick-weight-loss methods: fad diets and drugs.

Fad diets are usually very low-calorie diets—about 800 or less. Fad diets include: low-carbohydrate diet; high-carbohydrate diet; starvation or fasting diet; and protein-sparing modified fasts. Nutritionally inadequate diets may pose problems—particularly for MVPers who can experience changes in circulating blood volume, changes in sodium regulation, as well as changes in the autonomic nervous system.

Losses of sodium and water initially cause rapid weight loss—as much as 60% to 70%. For example, during a fasting or starvation diet, you can lose four to eight pounds within 24 hours. Also, when you initially fast, your sympathetic nervous-system activity increases and sometimes increases MVPS symptoms.

Next, when you severely reduce your caloric intake, your body thinks it's starving—which it is. To compensate, your body slows its metabolism, and defeats your original purpose—to drastically reduce calories. Furthermore, your metabolism may remain low for some time once you resume normal eating habits. Not only will you gain the weight back, but you also may become even heavier. Furthermore, without exercise, you lose water, fat, and muscle. You re-gain only fat and water. So what happens? You now replace active muscle tissue with inactive fat tissue, and slow your metabolism. Now, it becomes even *more difficult* to lose weight next time.

Something else changes: the renin-angiotensin-aldosterone system, which is a sodium-regulating mechanism. With inadequate food intake, the system may become less active and this causes sodium loss. In addition to lowering circulating blood volume, this low-sodium state may lead to an increase in sympathetic nervous system activity with an increase in MVPS symptoms.

To make matters worse, some diets require diet pills. These often are thyroid or water pills. Thyroid pills can increase the actions of many bodily functions. For instance, they can cause tachycardia (increased heart rate), nervousness, irritability, and increased bowel motility. Diuretics (water pills) reduce the circulating blood volume. The ill effects of these pills, therefore, initiate or worsen MVPS symptoms.

Do know that extreme diets don't often lead to changes in food habits that support a permanent weight loss. To lose weight, you must **BURN MORE CALORIES THAN YOU CONSUME**. To safely accomplish this, moderately reduce calories, consume required nutrients, and get regular cardiovascular exercise.

Simple Carbohydrates—Sugar

Why, and how, should I limit my intake of sugar?

Increased caloric intake, particularly from simple carbohydrates, sometimes increases MVPS symptoms. In fact, most calls to health care providers occur during the holidays. Why? Because holidays provide an excuse to indulge ourselves with pies, cakes, cookies, and candies.

When you consume sugar, especially by itself and not with a meal, there's an abrupt rise in blood glucose—blood sugar. This rise in blood glucose stimulates the secretion of insulin—the feasting hormone. Insulin stores glucose in the body's cells and lowers blood glucose. The decrease in blood glucose can stimulate epinephrine (adrenalin). The release of adrenalin can cause an increase in MVPS symptoms. It's not unusual, therefore, to hear MVPers complain of chest pains and extra beats following a mid-afternoon candy bar.

This doesn't mean that you need to totally cut sugar from your diet. Instead, fill up on nutrient-dense foods and then have an *occasional* sweet treat.

Continue to read food and beverage labels. To most people sugar is only refined white table sugar. There are, however, many sources of sugars. Any substance that ends with -*ose* is a sugar—sucrose is table sugar, lactose is milk sugar, and fructose is fruit sugar. Sugar is also found in processed foods such as soups, spaghetti sauces, fruit drinks, cereals, and yogurts. Too, sugar occurs naturally in fruits, vegetables, and dairy products.

Always study the ingredient list on food packages. Items are listed by weight in *descending order* according to their content. Therefore, be careful if sugar is listed first. This product contains a higher content of sugar than one in which sugar is listed *at the end* of the label. Beware that many manufactures call sugar by several different names. The amount of sugar in a product is sometimes misleading. For example, a granola cereal may have rolled oats listed first, brown sugar second, corn syrup third and honey fifth. Since *all* of these are sugars, sugar makes up most of this product.

TABLE 4-5. TEASPOONS OF SUGAR IN COMMON FOODS

Food	Serving Size	Teaspoons Sugar
Chewing gum	1 stick	1/2
Gingersnaps	1 medium	1
Marshmallow	1 average	1-1/2
Jam	1 tablespoon	3
Honey	1 tablespoon	3
Hamburger bun	1 bun	3
Caramel	3 pieces	4
Lowfat yogurt, plain	1 cup	4
Tang	8 ounces	4
Fruit cocktail	1/2 cup	5
Angel food cake	1/12 cake	6
Kool-Aid	8 ounces	6
Sherbet	1/2 cup	6–8
Soft drink	12 ounces	6–9
Apple pie	1/6 medium pie	12
Lowfat yogurt, fruited	1 cup	13
Chocolate cake, iced	1/12 cake	15

Sources: Brody, J. (1987). *Jane Brody's nutrition book.* New York: Bantam Books. Pennington, J., & Church, H. (1989). *Food values of portions commonly used.* (15th ed.). Philadelphia: J.B. Lippincott Co.

Avoid concentrated sugars, but not not fructose and lactose. Resist the temptation to snack on candy bars, pastries, and doughnuts—especially by themselves. If you crave M&M's or a Reese's cup, first eat a well-balanced meal. *Then* eat a sugary treat. Why? Nutrients such as fat, protein, and complex carbohydrates take longer to digest than sugar does. Therefore, your blood sugar may remain more stable than if you ate a concentrated, sugary food by itself.

Reduce sugar in baking. For example, sugar usually can be reduced by 1/3 and it won't affect the recipe. To add flavor, experiment with spices such as: cinnamon, cardamon, coriander, nutmeg, ginger, and mace. Avoid soft drinks or sodas. Prefer water with a piece of lemon or lime. Choose fruit for dessert. Fruit has a high water content and few calories. Use fructose instead of sucrose (table sugar). Fructose is 70% sweeter than sucrose, and you don't need as much.

Glycemic Index

More than 20 years ago, it was reported that simple sugars (i.e., mono- and disaccharides) were quickly digested and absorbed, thus causing a rapid and substantial rise in postprandial (after a meal) blood glucose (sugar). In contrast, complex carbohydrates (i.e., starches) were believed to be digested and absorbed more slowly and to have a more modest impact on blood glucose. Current available evidence, however, contradicts these beliefs. That is, the effects of carbohydrates on health are better described on the basis of their physiological effects, or the ability to raise blood glucose levels. This ability depends on a variety of factors such as the constituent of the sugar, the physical form of the carbohydrate, nature of the starch and other food components. Thus, the Food and Agriculture Organization (FAO) and the World Health Organization (WHO) recommend adopting the concept of "glycemic carbohydrate." Glycemic carbohydrates refer to the glycemic index (GI) and glycemic load (GL). Both the quality and quantity of carbohydrate determines an individual's glycemic response to a food or meal.

The glycemic index (GI) is a measure that ranks carbohydrate-containing foods according to their blood sugar response. That is, from this index, one can predict the rise in blood sugar two hours after a particular meal. A high-GI food (>70) with an equivalent carbohydrate content as a low-GI food (<55) produces a greater insulin response. Thus, high-GI foods may result in a lower blood sugar concentration 2-3 hours after a meal, where as a low-GI food results in a more steady glucose response.

The glycemic load (GL) provides a summary measure of the relative glycemic impact of a *typical* serving of a food. It is a weighted average glycemic index of foods and is the product of a food's GI and its total available carbohydrate content. For example, an apple has a GI value of approximately 40. A serving (medium-size apple) contains approximately 15 grams of carbohydrate. The glycemic load of an apple is: (40 × 15) divided by

100 = 6. Foods with a GL <10 are considered as low, >20 as high. For instance, a carrot has a high glycemic index, but a low glycemic load, in contrast to a potato, which has both a high GI and GL. In general, most refined starch foods have a high glycemic index, whereas non-starch vegetables, fruit, and legumes tend to have a low glycemic index. *(For glycemic charts, please see websites at the end of the chapter.)*

A few words of caution. Unfortunately, glycemic index is not that simple: Glycemic indexes of foods vary depending on the kind of food, its ripeness, the length of time it was stored, how it was cooked, its variety, and how it was processed; GI of a food varies from person to person and even in a single individual from day to day, depending on blood glucose levels, insulin resistance, and other factors. The GI of a food might be one value when it is eaten alone and another when it is eaten with other foods as part of a complete meal; and GI value is based on a portion that contains 50 grams of carbohydrate, which is rarely the amount typically eaten. Lastly, do not use the GL in isolation; doing so may lead to the habitual consumption of a lower-carbohydrate diet. The simplest way to consume a moderately high-carbohydrate, but low-GI diet is to follow the 2005 Dietary Guidelines for Americans (http://www.health.gov/dietaryguidelines).

Why are glycemic carbohydrates important? Reducing the rate of carbohydrate absorption by lowering the GI of your diet may have several health benefits. Chronic hyperglycemia (increased blood sugar) is a well known risk factor for cardiovascular disease and for the development of diabetes. Too, for MVPers, a lower GI may improve symptom control. Eating foods with a lower glycemic index may reduce insulin demand, improve blood sugar control, and reduce blood lipid (fat) concentrations. Incorporating a low-GI diet with other dietary interventions such as a high-fiber and low-saturated-fat diet with adequate amounts of micronutrients and fluids, may prove to have health benefits and help to control MVPS symptoms.

Satisfying that Sweet Tooth

Do you have a sweet tooth? Can't live without that chocolate bar? Then try these sweet recipes. They use little or no sugar, and are lower in saturated fat. For other recipes, see the references listed at the end of this chapter.

Flavorful Yogurt

INGREDIENTS:

> 8 ounces plain nonfat or lowfat yogurt
> 1 capful of vanilla or almond extract
> sweetener to taste—such as 2–3 packets of Nutrasweet
> 1/4 cup fresh chopped fruit (optional) such as straw-
> berries or peaches

DIRECTIONS: Mix all ingredients together. Refrigerate or freeze. Great as a snack or dessert. Serves 1.

Simple Apple Treat

INGREDIENTS:

> 1 apple cored, peeled, and sliced
> cinnamon to taste (about 1/8 teaspoon)
> dash of nutmeg (optional)
> sweetener (optional)

DIRECTIONS: Place sliced apples on a microwave-safe plate. Sprinkle cinnamon and a dash of nutmeg on top (optional). Cook in the microwave 3–5 minutes on high power till the desired consistency. Add sweetener such as Nutrasweet (optional). Serves 1.

Granola Apple Crisp

INGREDIENTS:

> 6 medium apples, peeled, cored, and sliced
> 1 tablespoon whole wheat flour
> 3/4 teaspoon cinnamon
> 1/4 teaspoon ground nutmeg
> 3/4 cup apple juice
> 1/4 cup packed brown sugar
> 3 tablespoons whole wheat flour
> 1/4 teaspoon cinnamon
> 1/4 teaspoon salt
> 1/4 cup margarine
> 1/2 cup quick or old-fashioned oats
> 3 tablespoon bran-type cereal or wheat germ
> 3 tablespoon chopped walnuts or pecans
> 1 teaspoon toasted sesame seeds

DIRECTIONS: In a bowl, stir together apples, 1 tablespoon flour, 3/4 teaspoon cinnamon, and 1/4 teaspoon nutmeg. Turn into an 8 × 8 × 2 baking dish. Build up edges slightly. Pour apple juice over fruit.

In another bowl, combine brown sugar, remaining flour, 1 teaspoon each of cinnamon and salt. Cut in margarine until well blended. Stir in remaining ingredients and sprinkle over fruit in center. Leave a ring of apples showing around edge.

Bake at 375° for 30 minutes. Serves 8.

Recipe reprinted with permission from the Greater Cincinnati Nutrition Council's Cookbook, *Nutritious and Delicious*, 1985.

Raspberry Cheesecake

INGREDIENTS:
  Pre-made graham cracker crust
  1 package sugar-free raspberry flavored gelatin
  1 cup boiling water
  1 container (16 ounces) lowfat cottage cheese
  1 cup part skim ricotta cheese
  2 cups fresh raspberries

DIRECTIONS: Stir sugar-free raspberry gelatin and boiling water until completely dissolved. Set aside until lukewarm. In a blender or food processor, blend cottage and ricotta cheeses until smooth; pour into large bowl. Blend in reserved gelatin mixture. Pour filling into crust. Chill until almost firm (about 3 hours). Top with 2 cups of raspberries. Chill at least 2 more hours. Serves 12.

Baked Banana

Place a whole ripe *unpeeled* banana on a cookie sheet. Bake at 350° for 20 minutes. Split the banana with knife; sprinkle with cinnamon or nutmeg.

Sugarless Cookies

INGREDIENTS:
  1-3/4 cups flour
  2 teaspoons baking powder
  1/2 teaspoon salt
  1/2 teaspoon cinnamon
  3/4 cup orange juice
  1/2 teaspoon grated orange rind
  1/2 cup minus 1 tablespoon vegetable oil
  1 egg
  1/2 cup chopped walnuts
  1/2 cup raisins

Directions: Preheat oven to 375°. Combine dry ingredients. Add remaining ingredients; mix well. Drop by teaspoon on ungreased cooking sheet to make 32–34 cookies. Bake about 15 to 20 minutes. When done, remove from pan and cool.

Variations: Add 1/4 teaspoon ground cloves for a spice drop. Instead of raisins, add 1/2 cup chopped or whole cranberries.

Source: *Family Cookbook.* Volume I. (1987). The American Diabetes Association and The American Dietetic Association.

Foods and Migraines

Why and How May Foods Possibly Trigger Migraines?

Migraines can be triggered by food, as well as a combination of other factors. It's believed that natural and artificial biochemicals contained within foods trigger headaches. For example, some migraine sufferers are deficient in the enzyme that digests amines. Therefore, any foods that contain the amino acid tyramine—or other amines—may cause migraines.

It's believed that tyramine acts either directly, or indirectly, through the release of norepinephrine—a powerful vasoconstrictor. Norepinephrine affects sensitive blood vessels that can cause a migraine attack. You'll find tyramine in foods and beverages such as cheddar and bleu cheese, and red wines that undergo bacterial decomposition.

Also, migraines can be triggered by eating foods containing nitrites such as hot dogs, bacon, sausage, and ham—cured meats. Additives, such as monosodium glutamate (MSG) found in some TV dinners and in some foods from Chinese restaurants, can also trigger migraines. Furthermore, eating high-fat meals may also trigger migraine headache. Many others who suffer with migraines must learn to recognize and avoid foods to which they are sensitive.

As a precautionary measure, avoid foods containing amines. Instead of aged cheeses such as Swiss, cheddar or provolone, choose ricotta, cottage or American cheese. If red wine, brandy or beer trigger a migraine, drink white wine. Choose freshly prepared meat rather than canned or aged ham, bacon, sausage, hot dogs or dried fish. If yeast breads—white or sourdough breads—trigger an attack, eat whole wheat and rye breads. Avoid high-fat meals; decrease fat intake to 20% of total daily calories.

Natural products that may be effective in the treatment of migraine headaches include feverfew (*Tanacetum parthenium*), riboflavin (400 mg), butterbur (*Petasites hybridus* root) (75 mg twice daily), and coenzyme Q10. In addition, alternative therapies such as acupuncture and chiropractic manipulation may be helpful in the treatment and prevention of migraines.

Keep a food diary. Then, see what you ate *prior* to each migraine attack. Try to identify the culprits. Avoid them for a trial period of time, and see what happens.

Magnesium Intake

Why and How May a Magnesium Deficiency Possibly Affect Me?

As mentioned in Chapter 1, there's evidence that magnesium deficiency may play a role in MVPS symptoms. Therefore, avoid diets high in fats. Fat substances inhibit the absorption of magnesium. Dietary phosphates—very high in certain sodas—also inhibit reabsorption of magnesium. Study the following chart, and limit your intake of soft drinks high in phosphates.

Refining foods, especially white sugar and grains, causes large losses of magnesium. In cooking and baking, substitute brown sugar for white. One-half cup of brown sugar contains 20 milligrams of magnesium; white sugar has none. Steam—don't boil vegetables—to preserve magnesium.

MVPers should get an adequate amount of magnesium daily—420 mg for men, 360 mg for women—by eating a well-balanced diet. Good sources of magnesium include nuts, legumes, cereal, grains, green leafy vegetables, apples, apricots, avocados, bananas, blackstrap molasses, brewer's yeast, brown rice, figs, garlic, kelp, lima beans, peaches, wheat and whole grains.

As MVPers, exercise caution, and *never assume that you're deficient in magnesium. Don't take supplements without first consulting your health care provider.* Magnesium supplements may be unnecessary, or even forbidden, as for example, with impaired kidney function.

On the other hand, provided magnesium supplements are advised, consider the following facts. Oral magnesium supplements combine magnesium with another substance such as a salt. Examples of magnesium supplements include magnesium oxide, magnesium sulfate, and magnesium carbonate. Elemental magnesium refers to the amount of magnesium in each compound: magnesium oxide has the greatest amount and

TABLE 4-6. SELECTED FOOD SOURCES OF MAGNESIUM[a]

FOOD	Milligrams (mg)	%DV
Halibut, cooked, 3 ounces	90	20
Almonds, dry roasted, 1 ounce	80	20
Cashews, dry roasted, 1 ounce	75	20
Soybeans, mature, cooked, ½ cup	75	20
Spinach, frozen, cooked, ½ cup	75	20
Nuts, mixed, dry-roasted, 1 ounce	65	15
Cereal, shredded wheat, 2 rectangular biscuits	55	15
Oatmeal, instant, fortified, prepared w/water, 1 cup	55	15
Potato, baked w/ skin, 1 medium	50	15
Peanuts, dry-roasted, 1 ounce	50	15
Peanut butter, smooth, 2 tablespoons	50	15
Wheat bran, crude, 2 tablespoons	45	10
Black-eyed peas, cooked, ½ cup	45	10
Yogurt, plain, skim milk, 8 fluid ounces	45	10
Bran flakes, ¾ cup	40	10
Vegetarian baked beans, ½ cup	40	10
Rice, brown, long-grained, cooked, ½ cup	40	10
Lentils, mature seeds, cooked, ½ cup	35	8
Avocado, California, ½ cup pureed	35	8
Kidney beans, canned, ½ cup	35	8
Pinto beans, cooked, ½ cup	35	8
Wheat germ, crude, 2 tablespoons	35	8
Chocolate milk, 1 cup	33	8
Banana, raw, 1 medium	30	8
Milk chocolate candy bar, 1.5 ounce bar	28	8
Milk, reduced fat (2%) or fat-free, 1 cup	27	8
Bread, whole wheat, commercially prepared, 1 slice	25	6
Raisins, seedless, ¼ cup packed	25	6
Whole milk, 1 cup	24	6
Chocolate pudding, 4-ounce ready-to-eat portion	24	6

[a]DV = Daily value. For foods not listed in this table, please refer to the U.S. Department of Agriculture's Nutrient Database Web site: http://www.nal.usda.gov/fnic/cgi-bin/nut_search.pl.

Source: U.S. Department of Agriculture, Agricultural Research Service. 2003. USDA National Nutrient Database for Standard Reference, Release 16. Nutrient Data Laboratory Home Page: http://www.nal.usda.gov/fnic/foodcomp.

magnesium sulfate the least. The amount of elemental magnesium in a compound and its bioavailability influence the effectiveness of the magnesium supplement. (Bioavailability refers to the degree of a drug's availability to the body's tissues after administration.) Enteric coating of a magnesium compound can decrease bioavailability. Older studies suggest that magnesium oxide has a lower bioavailability while magnesium chloride and magnesium lactate have significantly higher and equal absorption and bioavailability. However, recent reformulation of certain magnesium oxide preparations to improve solubility and to meet the standards of the U.S. Pharmocopeia have improved bioavailability. Oral magnesium supplements sometimes cause gastrointestinal side effects such as nausea and diarrhea. In this situation, consider dividing your dose in half and taking your supplement with your largest meal for the first few weeks. Recommended oral magnesium therapy ranges from 400–600 mg. Avoid doses higher than 800 mg per day.

Non-prescription Drugs

The Negative Effects of Some Non-prescription Drugs

Caffeine is not limited to foods and beverages. There are over 1000 prescription medications and over 2000 non-prescription, or OTC (over-the-counter) drugs that contain caffeine. These caffeine levels widely vary. Typical caffeine-containing prescription drugs contain 30–100 mg caffeine per tablet or capsule, while OTC drugs contain a wider range—up to 200 mg or more per tablet. Read labels. Obtain information from your pharmacist.

Do some contain other stimulants that may worsen my symptoms?

There are many non-prescription drugs that contain ephedrine and pseudoephedrine. Ephedrine and pseudoephedrine stimulate the sympathetic system and may worsen MVPS symptoms. Examples include: Actified, Benadryl, Chlor-Trimeton, Drixoral antihistamine, Congestac, CoTylenol, Novahistine DMX, Robitussin-PE, Sinutab, Sine-Aid, Tylenol Maximum Strength and Sudafed. (For information on antihistamines and decongestants, see Chapter 9.) Avoid medications that contain adrenalin and adrenalin-like substances.

OTC Preparations	Caffeine (mg/tablet)
Stimulants	
NoDoz	100
Vivarin	200
Pain Relievers	
Anacin	32
Excedrin	65
Excedrin P.M.	0
Midol	32
Vanquish	33
Appetite Suppressants	
Dexatrim	200
Ma Huang (caffeine & herbal ephedra)	150
Cold Remedies	
Coryban-D	30
Dristan	32
Neo-synephrine	15
Sinarest	30
Triaminicin	33

SOURCE: FDA's Center for Drugs and Biologics

References

Aufderheide, S., D. Lax & S.J. Goldberg. 1995. Gender differences in dehydration-induced mitral valve prolapse. *American Heart Journal* **129**(1): 83–86.

Balch, J. & P. Balch, P. 1990. Prescription for Nutritional Healing. Avery Publishing Group, Inc. Garden City Park, NY.

Barclay, Alan W., Jennie C. Brand-Miller & Thomas M.S. Wolever. 2005. Glycemic index, glycemic load, and glycemic response are not the same. *Diabetes Care* **28**(7): 1839–1840.

Brewed Coffee. October, 1994. *Consumer Reports* **69**: 640–651.

Colombani, Paolo C. 2004. Glycemic index and load-dynamic dietary guidelines in the context of diseases. *Physiology & Behavior* **83**(4): 603–610.

Dietary Reference Intakes for Water, Potassium, Sodium, Chloride, and Sulfate. 2004. Panel on Dietary Reference Intakes for Electrolytes and Water, Standing Committee on the Scientific Evaluation of Dietary Reference Intakes. National Academies Press. Available at http://www.nap.edu/catalog/10925.html

Fine, K., C. Santa Ana, J. Porter & J.S. Fordtran. 1991. Intestinal absorption of magnesium from food and supplements. *Journal of Clinical Investigation* **88**(2): 396–402.

Firoz, M. & M. Graber. 2001. Bioavailaility of US commercial magnesium preparation. *Magnesium Res.* **14:** 257–62.

Freedman, M., J. King & E. Kennedy. 2001. Popular diets: A scientific review. *Obesity Research* **9** (suppl): 1S–40S.

Freeman, R. 2003. Treatment of orthostatic hypotension. *Seminars in Neurology* **23**(4): 435–442.

Gaffney, F. & C. Blomqvist. 1988. Mitral valve prolapse and autonomic nervous system dysfunction: A pathophysiological link. *In* Mitral Valve Prolapse and the Mitral Valve Prolapse Syndrome. H. Boudoulas & C. Wooley, Eds. pp. 427–443. Futura Publishing Co. New York.

Galland, L., S. Baker & R. McLellan. 1986. Magnesium deficiency in the pathogenesis of mitral valve prolapse. *Magnesium* **5:** 165–174.

Klasco, R.K., Ed. 2003. USP DI® Drug Information for the Healthcare Professional. Thomson MICROMEDEX. Greenwood Village, Colorado.

Klein, M. 1994. Magnesium therapy in cardiovascular disease. *Cardiovascular Review and Report.* pp. 9-27.

Kleiner, S. 1999. Water: An essential but overlooked nutrient. *Journal of the American Dietetic Association* **99:** 200–206.

Latzka, W.A. & J. Montain. 1999. Water and electrolyte requirements for exercise. *Clinics in Sports Medicine* **18**(3), 513–524.

Lax, D., M. Eicher & S.J. Goldberg. 1993. Effects of hydration on mitral valve prolapse. *American Heart Journal* **126**(2): 415–418.

Lax, D., M. Eicher & S.J. Goldberg. 1992. Mild dehydration induces echocardiographic signs of mitral valve prolapse in healthy females with prior normal cardiac findings. *American Heart Journal* **124**(6): 1533–1540.

Ludwign, D. 2002. The glycemic index: Physiology mechanisms relating to obesity, diabetes, and cardiovascular disease. *JAMA* **287:** 2414–2423.

Maughan, R. & J. Griffin, J. 2003. Caffeine ingestion and fluid balance: A review. *Journal of Human Nutrition and Dietetics* **16:** 411–420.

Opperman, A. M. *et al.* 2004. Meta-analysis of the health effects of using the glycaemic index in meal-planning. *The British Journal of Nutrition* **92**(3): 367–381.

Pennington, J. & H. Church. 1985. Food Values of Portions Commonly Used, 14th ed. Harper & Row Publishers. New York.

Shirreffs, S.M. & J. Maughan. 1997. Restoration of fluid balance after exercise-induced dehydration: effects of alcohol consumption. *Journal of Applied Physiology* **83**(4): 1152–1158.

Silberstein, S. 2004. Migraine. *The Lancet* **363:** 381–391.

Solomon, S. 1991. The Headache Book. Consumer Reports Books.

Winkelmayer, M., M. Stampfer, W. Willett, *et al.* 2005. Habitual caffeine intake and the risk of hypertension in women. *JAMA* **294:** 2330–2335.

5

The Positive Effects of Mind Over Matter

Move It

Can you identify with this scenario? As you sit and watch TV, or as you sit at a desk, you suddenly feel a flip-flop sensation from those nasty extra beats. "I'm having a heart attack. I *know* this time it's fatal," you say to yourself.

What do you do? You take your pulse. One skipped beat, two skipped beats, three skipped beats. "Oh no, this IS it."

And what do you keep doing? You continue to sit, and you continue to take your pulse. Your sense of fear intensifies and makes matters worse. You become even more frightened. Your nervous system releases more and more adrenalin. Now, the chest pains begin. What can I do?

Don't sit. Don't panic. Don't take your pulse. Instead, *move it.* Get up; get busy; or take a walk. As you do, your heart rate increases and usually overrides—or suppresses—extra beats. Furthermore, when you're busy you re-focus your energies *on the task and not on the extra heartbeats.*

Janet, one of our program participants, who formerly sat, checked her pulse and panicked when she experienced extra beats, followed our advice. Now, every time she feels extra beats, she vacuums.

"This idea works," she said, "and I also have the cleanest house in town."

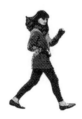

Pursed-lip Breathing

Can pursed-lip breathing help to overcome shortness of breath?

Pursed-lip breathing effectively helps many MVPers overcome their inability to take a deep breath. Therefore, whenever you feel breathless, take a breath—any kind—whether it's short or deep through your nose. Next, *slowly* breathe out through your mouth with your lips pursed—as if you're blowing out a candle. Don't breathe out through your nose.

Again, take a breath—a deeper one. To exhale, repeat. Breathe out *slowly* through pursed lips.

Repeat the cycle till you can take full, deep breaths. Remember to always *breathe out slowly* through pursed lips and after three or four breaths, you should feel relief.

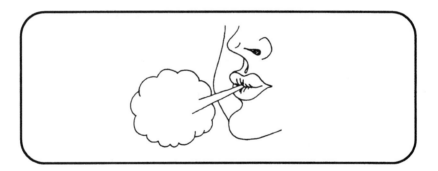

Feet Up

Which techniques can I use to help relieve chest pains associated with MVPS?

Lie down on your back and bend your knees, or raise your legs. Place your legs either on a couch or against the wall. The chest pain often subsides within a few minutes.

Of course, this isn't always feasible, particularly if you're at work or in a crowded shopping mall. Here's a variation. Sit crossed-legged (Indian style) and lean your head forward toward your knees.

Do know that these techniques *are not* appropriate treatments for chest pains caused by other medical conditions.

Exercise

Because exercise is a *key factor* in reducing the frequency, intensity and severity of MVPS symptoms, it is discussed in detail in the next chapter.

Stress and Mindfulness Meditation

Does stress exacerbate MVPS symptoms, and can I be helped through mindfulness meditation?

Daily living causes both outer and inner stressors. Typical outer stressors result from people stress, time stress, and role stress. Inner stressors, on the other hand, relate to physical, mental, and emotional states such as fatigue, obsessive thinking, and anxiety or depression.

If stressors cause a significant stress reaction and increase activity of the autonomic nervous system (ANS), *yes*, they may activate or even worsen MVPS symptoms. And no drugs by themselves provide immunity to stress or pain and solve life's problems.

Each one of us must realize the futility of expecting *someone else* to make things better. Although some forces are beyond our control, others really are not. To a great extent, *we* influence circumstances by the way we see things. How we see things determines how much energy we have and how we positively channel that energy in the right direction. Such energy comes from inside, is within our reach, and is within our potential control. How can we tap into it? Cultivate mindfulness meditation and discover deep realms of relaxation, calmness, and insight.

What, then, is mindfulness meditation? Mindfulness is an ancient practice of being in the present moment fully and feeling each moment as a new beginning. It is a way of paying attention, a way of looking deeply within oneself to gain understanding. There is a way to look at problems, to come to terms with problems, and to make life more joyful *when you are in control.* This is a way of being, a way of awareness, a way of mindfulness. Unlike familiar forms of meditation that involve focusing on a sound, a phrase, or a prayer to minimize distracting thoughts, mindfulness recommends the opposite. Rather than ignore distracting thoughts, sensations, or physical discomfort—focus on them.

As an MVPer, challenge your mindfulness. Say to yourself, "Right now I live my life, and I make many choices. In a stressful situation, I *choose* to react; or I *choose* to calmly respond."

Therefore, whenever you're stressed, don't feel helpless or adopt a fight-or-flight solution. Instead, let mindfulness—moment-to-moment awareness—help you to take control. Increase your level of awareness and decide *how* to manage it for the better.

To do so, bring your awareness to your face and shoulders as they tense up, to your heart as it pounds, to your lungs if you're breathless, or to any other needy part of your body. Again, say to yourself, "I *choose* to overcome it."

Next, focus on your breath. Your breath reconnects you with calmness, and brings you to an awareness of your whole body. To meditate, *feel* the movement of air as it flows in and out past your nostrils. *Feel* the movement of your chest as it expands and contracts. Don't push or force each breath. Simply *be aware* of its feeling. As you do so, with each breath you center not on the past nor in the future. You center on the *present* moment. Your mind and your body unite in the present.

NOTE: Although you learn to respond to stress with awareness, it doesn't mean you'll never react or become overwhelmed by anger, grief, or fear. Instead, you'll gradually learn how to control and how to deal with stress. The idea isn't to suppress your emotions, but to learn how to control and deal with them. To respond to stress requires moment-to-moment awareness. Take each moment as it comes.

Body-scan Meditation

Following a hectic day, use the body scan before retiring. Lie on your back and focus your mind throughout different regions of your body. Begin with the toes of one foot, up the leg to the pelvis and feel the sensations as you direct your breath to and from each region. Repeat the procedures on the other foot and leg. Next, direct your breath to remaining parts of your body till you reach the top of your head. End up by breathing through an imaginary hole in the top of your head. Throughout the scan as you imagine the placement of each breath, also imagine feelings of fatigue and tension as they flow out each time you exhale. Believe that each *new* breath brings vitality and relaxation.

Sitting Meditation

Sit in a comfortable position and focus on your breath. Soon your attention wanders to various thoughts, feelings, or body sensations. With this practice you note thoughts, feelings and body sensations, but you don't dwell on them. Instead, you direct your attention to your breathing. Use sitting mediation upon arising to clear your mind, center your thoughts, and give you renewed clarity and energy.

Walking Meditation

Enjoy a walk with nowhere to go, no time to be there. Fully experience your body as you walk on earth during this time. Take purposeful steps, placing your heel and then your toes on the ground. Feel the earth beneath you.

Mindful Hatha Yoga

Another technique helpful in lessening MVPS symptoms is mindful hatha yoga—gentle stretching and strengthing exercises, with moment-to-moment awareness of breathing and bodily sensations during various postures. As one program participant says, "Through yoga, I learned how to relax, and how to breathe. I learned that you can't relax till you're breathing correctly. It takes time to learn, but the time is well spent. I also know that not every bodily sensation is MVPS-related. Now, I can deal with these sensations—and not panic. Before learning yoga, I did. Yoga helped me effectively deal with my MVPS symptoms, and I'm more at peace with myself."

A complete description of mindfulness training is beyond the scope of this chapter. If interested in learning more about these practices, see references listed at the end of the chapter. In addition, check your local newspaper for meditation programs.

Tangible Feedback

The Benefits Derived from Tangible Feedback

Why should I monitor my progress with a symptom check list?

Now that you're aware of interventions that help to control MVPS symptoms, monitor your progress with the *symptom check list*. It was originally developed for a research study. The check list was used to monitor symptoms of MVPS on a weekly basis, and to note changes over time. Since its development, many MVPers used the symptom check list to assess their progress. It's one way to note your improvements.

Take a moment now and complete the check list. Think of the past week. Which symptoms did you experience, and how frequent were they? If you experienced chest pain every day, place a five in the frequency column opposite chest pain. If you had palpitations or extra beats one or two times for the entire week, then place a one next to this symptom.

Start using the non-drug interventions you've learned. At the end of each week, fill out this check list. Do this for twelve weeks. You'll be pleased at how well you do.

Next, take a piece of graph paper and plot the frequency numbers for each symptom over 12 weeks. On the left-hand side of the graph write the numbers 0 to 5—or 0 to 3 if you never had higher than a 3. On the bottom, write the weeks 1 to 12. What you'll see is an overall decrease in the frequency of your symptoms.

The following example is from a research study done at the MVPPC. The weekly average of the frequency for the symptom *mood swings* for the exercise group and the control group—non-exercise group—are plotted over 12 weeks. Note the difference

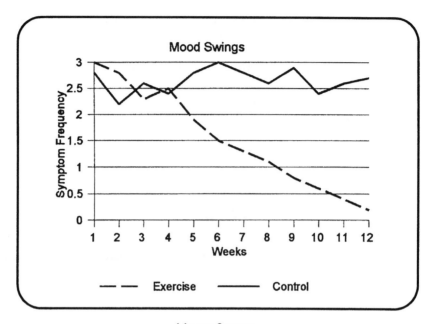

MOOD SWINGS

between the two groups, and the decrease in frequency of mood swings in the exercise group.

Another idea is a behavioral chart developed by an MVPer. Use this chart in combination with the symptom check list.

Behavior	Poor	Fair	Good	Excellent
Sugar intake				
Caffeine intake				
Water intake				
Sodium intake				
Exercise				
Stress				
Personal schedule				

Submitted by: M. Goodwin, Belleville, Illinois. 1992.

If you're eating lots of chocolate or other sweets, then check poor for sugar and caffeine intake. In other words, you did a poor job of following advice for symptom control. If you feel under lots of stress, then mark poor next to stress. If you over-booked yourself—many places to go and not enough time—mark poor next to personal schedule.

SYMPTOM CHECK LIST

Name_____ Week #____ Week ending ___/___/___

Please place a number next to the symptom that best indicates the frequency
with which you experienced this symptom during the **past week:**

> 5—All of the time
> 4—Most of the time
> 3—A good bit of the time
> 2—Some of the time
> 1—A little of the time
> 0—None of the time

SYMPTOM	FREQUENCY
Chest pain and/or chest discomfort	
Arm pain and/or arm discomfort	
Palpitations/extra beats/skipped beats/heart pounding	
Shortness of breath	
Fatigue	
Headache	
Anxious (feeling nervous or frightened)	
Mood swings	
Dizziness and/or lightheadedness	
Passing out spells (losing consciousness)	
Muscle cramps	

I saw my physician ____Yes ____No. If yes, was this a routine visit?____Yes ____No.

I missed ____ days from work.

I went to the emergency room for treatment ____Yes ____No.

Selected References

Feuerstein, G. & Bodian, S. , Eds. 1993. Living Yoga: A Comprehensive Guide for Daily Life. Putnam Publishing Group. New York.

Kabat-Zinn, J. 1990. Full Catastrophe Living: Using the Wisdom of Your Body and Mind to Face Stress, Pain, and Illness. Delta. New York.

Kabat-Zinn, J., A. Massion, J. Kristeller *et al.* 1992. Effectiveness of a meditation-based stress reduction program in the treatment of anxiety disorders. *American Journal of Psychiatry* **149**: 936–943.

Scordo, K. 1991. Effects of aerobic exercise training on symptomatic women with mitral valve prolapse. *American Journal of Cardiology* **67**: 863–867.

Toseland, R. & R. Rivas.1984. An Introduction to Group Work Practice. Macmillan Publishing Co. New York.

Watkins, P. & R. Russell. 1990. Mitral valve prolapse syndrome 1990: Appropriate diagnosis is key to a happy patient. *Illustrated Medicine* **5:** 1–15.

6

Exercise and MVPS

"Exercise? I can hardly get out of bed in the morning."

"I have to conserve my limited energy."

"I have no time—I'm too busy."

"I'm afraid to exercise. Something terrible will happen."

Sound familiar? Some MVPers fear the consequences of exercise. Others fear a need to conserve limited energy. Do know inactivity causes deconditioning—an undoing of physical fitness. *Symptoms do not decrease with inactivity—they increase.*

Deconditioned people experience reduced exercise tolerance—they can't do as much, or last as long. Deconditioning causes symptoms similar to those of MVPS. It often becomes difficult to determine where the symptoms of deconditioning end and where the deconditioning symptoms of MVPS begin. For instance, as with MVPers, deconditioned people have high resting heart rates. This is analogous to racing a car's engine when it's idling. Then, with minimal activity, there is a rapid, inappropriate increase in heart rate. This causes shortness of breath, and feelings of fatigue that lead to further inactivity. Thus, the cycle continues. The less you do, the less you feel like doing. This cycle, however, can be broken with regular cardiovascular exercise.

Although regular cardiovascular exercise benefits many people, it particularly benefits MVPers (see list on next page). Those who regularly exercise have fewer symptoms and more endurance than those who don't.

Physical fitness not only helps you get the most out of life, it also helps equip you to meet everyday demands. Regardless of either your age or your present level of fitness, you'll benefit from a program of proper cardiovascular exercise.

**IMPORTANT CARDIOVASCULAR TRAINING EFFECTS:
BENEFITS FOR MVPERS**

- Lowered plasma catecholamines—epinephrine or adrenalin and norepinephrine—believed responsible for some MVPS symptoms
- Lowered resting heart rate
- Increased maximal cardiac output—the amount of blood the heart pumps in one minute at peak exercise
- Decrease in heart rate at any matched submaximal work load—lower heart rate while doing the same amount of work
- Increase in both maximal and submaximal stroke volume—the amount of blood pumped out of the heart's ventricles with each beat
- Increase in resting blood volume
- Improvement of stress management, reduction of the effects of stress, and a quicker recovery from psychosocial stress
- Increased alertness and self-confidence
- Increased endurance and energy level
- Promotion of a sense of well-being

What is Physical Fitness?

The President's Council on Physical Fitness and Sports defined physical fitness as "the ability to carry out daily tasks with vigor and alertness, without much fatigue, and with enough energy to enjoy leisure-time pursuits, and to meet unforeseen emergencies." In other words, you should have not only enough energy to survive, but enough energy to enjoy life.

COMPONENTS OF PHYSICAL FITNESS

- Cardiorespiratory fitness
- Flexibility
- Muscular fitness
- Body composition

The four components of physical fitness include:

(1) *Cardiorespiratory (aerobic) fitness:* the ability of the heart, lung, and circulatory system to take in, deliver, and use oxygen needed for cellular energy production. Aerobic fitness enhances endurance and lessens MVPS symptoms. (You may measure your level of cardiorespiratory fitness by a graded exercise stress test.)

(2) *Flexibility:* the maximum ability to move a joint through a range of motion. For example, the trunk flexion or sit-and-reach test evaluates hamstring and low back flexibility. Adequate flexibility is important for activities that require bending and stretching. Flexibility is also important for preventing injury and soreness during activities. MVPers often have increased joint flexibility.

(3) *Muscular fitness—two types of muscular fitness:* the first is muscular strength—the maximal force generated by a specific muscle or muscle group. For example, the heaviest weight you lift one time on a leg extension is the muscular strength of your quadriceps—the group of muscles in the front of your thigh. Activities such as carrying groceries or carrying small children require varying degrees of muscular strength.

The second type of muscular fitness is muscular endurance—the ability of a muscle group to exert a less-than-maximal force for an extended period of time. Exercises such as biking and rowing require muscular endurance.

(4) *Body composition:* the percentage of your weight that is fat. Body composition is more important than actual weight. For example, your weight might be within the proper range on a height-and-weight chart, but your percentage of body fat is high. Conversely, you might be overweight on the chart, but in actuality be slender and have good muscle tone. To calculate an ideal body weight, therefore, consider your body composition. Don't rely on only a height-and-weight chart.

Together, these components constitute overall physical fitness. Not every exercise, however, improves *all* of these components. For example, although doing house work, carrying groceries, and lifting weights are work, they are not considered cardiovascular exercise. Therefore, these activities lack the important symptom-controlling benefits of regular aerobic exercise.

Types of Exercise and Their Benefits

Aerobic Exercise

Aerobic means *with oxygen.* Aerobic (endurance) exercise uses oxygen to produce energy. Moderate in intensity, aerobic exercise involves the rhythmic movement of large muscle groups. This type of exercise conditions the cardiovascular system. Examples include bicycling, jogging, rowing, swimming, brisk walking, and cross-country skiing. Aerobic exercise also improves muscular endurance and body composition—two components of fitness. Fat is burned, muscle tone is increased, and body composition is improved.

Short Term (Acute) Effects of Aerobic Exercise

Acute effects of exercise include an increase in heart rate, stroke volume (the amount of blood the heart pumps each beat), and cardiac output (the amount of blood the heart pumps in a minute). These effects help meet the increased demand for oxygenated blood, and create additional energy required for exercise. Aerobically untrained MVPers, however, tend to have greater heart-rate increases than those aerobically untrained people *without* MVPS.

Exercise also affects blood pressure. Systolic blood pressure (upper number in a blood pressure reading) is the pressure in arteries when the heart contracts. Diastolic blood pressure (the lower number in a blood pressure reading) is the pressure in arteries between heart beats. Normally to meet the increased demand for blood, systolic pressure increases with activity and diastolic pressure remains the same.

Exercise also decreases circulating-stress hormones such as adrenalin and its related substances. Following exercise, you feel relaxed and more alert.

Training Effects of Aerobic Exercise

Training effects—long-term benefits—of regular aerobic exercise begin within six to eight weeks. By then, most MVPers notice a decrease in symptoms.

With cardiovascular training, your resting heart rate becomes lower and your heart rate's response to exercise improves. Now, when you climb a flight of stairs, your heart rate increases to only 90 beats per minute, instead of 150 beats as it did three months ago. In essence, you taught your cardiovascular system how to function more economically.

Intravascular blood volume and cardiac output increase with cardiovascular training. This helps alleviate the forceful heart beat and any feeling of lightheadedness when you stand up. Furthermore, blood levels of the adrenalin-like substances (catecholamines) may decrease. This may lessen the extra beats, chest pains, anxiety, and other MVPS symptoms.

Training effects also improve muscle tone, muscular endurance, and your body's response to other activities. But, these cardiovascular training effects last *only* if you continue regular exercise. Once you stop, you can lose the benefits of aerobic conditioning within two weeks. To receive continued benefits, therefore, plan to exercise throughout your lifetime.

Anaerobic Exercise

Anaerobic exercise, such as sprinting or strength training, is high-intensity exercise that uses glycogen—carbohydrates stored in the muscles. This type of exercise causes a rapid depletion of glycogen stores and the build-up of lactic acid. Although anaerobic exercise doesn't benefit the cardiovascular system, it does increase muscular strength—a component of fitness.

Types of Muscular Strength Training

(1) *Isotonic*—same tension: Isotonic contractions occur when a weight is held constant while the muscle shortens and lengthens. Examples of isotonic exercise include pushups, situps, lifting free weights and using weight stations such as Universal machines.

(2) *Isokinetic*—same movement: Isokinetic contractions occur as a muscle shortens to counteract a resistance developed by a special machine. The speed of the contraction remains constant and the resistance to the contraction remains proportional to the force exerted. In other words, the harder you push or pull, the more resistance you feel while the speed remains the same. You accomplish isokinetic muscle contractions with expensive mechanical equipment such as a Cybex dynamometer (Lumex, Bay Shore, NY). Competitive athletes use this equipment to improve their range of joint motion. Others use isokinetic exercise to rehabilitate injured muscles. For most people, however, isokinetic exercise equipment is unnecessary.

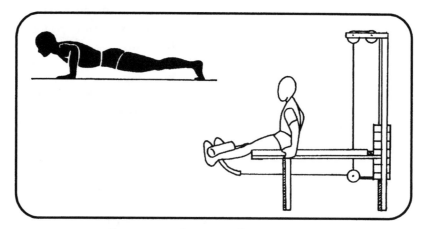

EXAMPLES OF ISOTONIC CONTRACTIONS

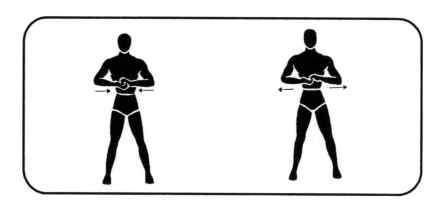

EXAMPLE OF ISOMETRIC CONTRACTIONS

(3) *Isometric*—same measure: Isometric (static) muscular contractions occur when muscular tension develops without much muscle movement. An example of an isometric contraction is pushing your hands together to create tension without moving your arms. Other examples include carrying heavy luggage, or carrying heavy bags of groceries. Isometric contractions can cause abrupt rises in blood pressure. Therefore, people with hypertension—high blood pressure—should avoid this type of strength training. Because of abrupt blood volume changes, isometric exercises should generally be avoided by MVPers.

> *The most important type of exercise for people with MVPS is aerobic exercise. This form of exercise produces the physiological adaptations that reduce the frequency and intensity of MVPS symptoms.*

The Exercise Prescription: Aerobic Exercise

Each exercise prescription is designed to enhance physical fitness, promote health, and ensure one's safety during participation. Exercise prescriptions vary with a person's interests, needs, background, and health status. The most desirable exercise prescription, however, helps you to habitually increase your physical activity and to decrease your MVPS symptoms. A discussion of the five components of an exercise prescription—intensity, mode, duration, frequency, and progression of physical activity—follows.

Warming Up

Warming up prepares your body for exercise in a number of ways. It does so by gradually increasing your heart rate, distributing blood to exercising muscles, warming the temperature of muscles, and improving circulation. Warming up decreases muscle soreness and decreases the risk of injury to muscles, tendons, ligaments and other connective tissues. Furthermore, warming up reduces muscle tightness and cramping.

To warm up for an aerobic activity, first walk around for a few minutes, and then perform slow stretches. Next, work at an intensity *of fairly light* on the rating of perceived exertion (RPE) scale. Keep your target heart rate below your target heart rate range (THR). Do this for at least five minutes. (RPE and THR ranges are discussed in later paragraphs.)

Cooling Down

Cooling down gradually decreases your heart rate and recirculates and redistributes blood. It is very important that MVPers properly cool down after exercise.

When exercise is abruptly stopped without cooling down, blood tends to pool in muscles that were exercised. For example, if you were walking or biking, blood would pool in your legs.

As blood pools, less blood recirculates throughout your body. MVPers tend to already have a lower blood volume, and therefore, less blood to circulate. Without proper cooling down, MVPers are more prone to lightheadedness, dizziness, and palpitations. Furthermore, cooling down decreases the risk of muscle soreness, injury, and fatigue. Therefore, cool down for a minimum of five to ten minutes. Perform your last exercise slowly. Do so at an RPE of *fairly light*. Example: If your last exercise is walking on a treadmill at 4.0 mph at a 5% grade, then walk at 0% and gradually decrease the speed. To finish, stretch the major muscle groups that you used.

Stretching

During your initial warmup and during the last part of your cool down, stretch all major muscles you either will use or did use in your workout activity. This must be done correctly.

To warm your muscles and maximize flexibility, walk for a few minutes prior to your warmup stretches. Hold each stretch for 10–20 seconds. Don't stretch beyond a feeling of a slight muscle pull. *Do not bounce.* Bouncing activates a muscular reflex—the stretch reflex. Instead of stretching, your muscles contract. Bouncing combined with contracting muscle can produce injury and soreness, and doesn't improve flexibility.

If you feel pain during the stretch, lessen the amount you are stretching. If pain persists, avoid that stretch. *Do not hold your breath*—breathe normally.

If your symptoms include lightheadedness or dizziness when standing up, avoid stretches that involve abrupt postural changes. These include windmills and touching the floor from a standing position.

Examples of Warmup and Cool Down Exercises

As you preform these stretches, hold the stretch to where you feel a slight pull in the muscle.

Do not bounce and do not hold your breath.

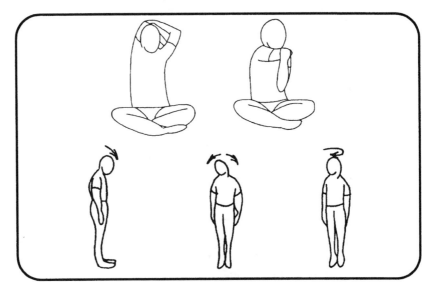

SHOULDER AND ARM STRETCHES

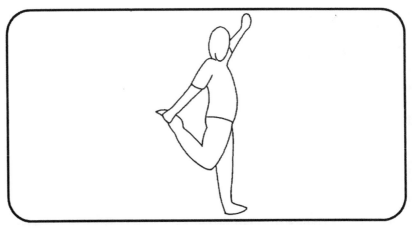

QUADRICEPS STRETCH: Pull your leg straight back until you feel a slight pull in your quadriceps—the muscles in front of your thigh. *Variation:* Do the same by lying on your side.

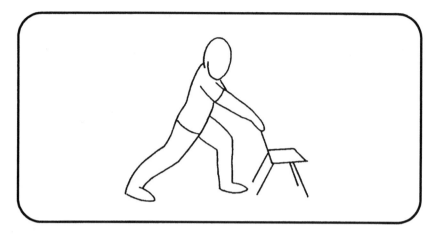

CALF STRETCH: Place one foot in front of the other. Point both feet straight forward, with your heels flat. Lunge forward with front leg bent and back leg straight.

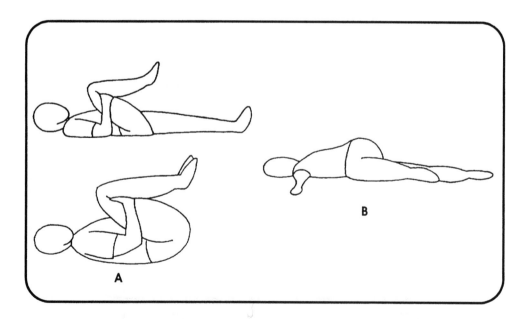

LOWER BACK STRETCHES: Stretches lower back and gluteal—buttock—muscles. Stretches lower back and hip muscles.

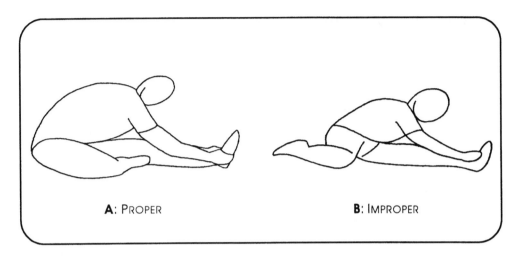

A: PROPER   **B**: IMPROPER

A. HAMSTRING STRETCH: Place one foot on the opposite knee. Keep your leg straight with foot pointed toward the ceiling. Bend forward from your waist till you feel a slight pull in your hamstrings—muscle on the back of your thigh.

B. IMPROPER HAMSTRING STRETCH: This can strain your knees.

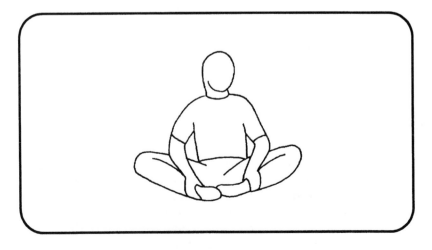

INNER LEG STRETCH

Exercises to Avoid with MVPS

Avoid exercises that involve abrupt postural changes such as the following:

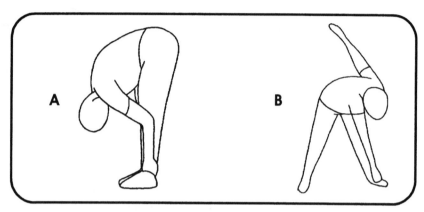

A. BENDING OVER TO TOUCH YOUR TOES.   B. WINDMILLS

Avoid activities requiring extreme exertion.

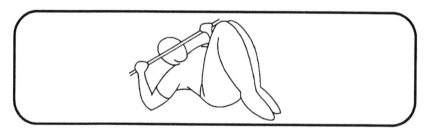

LIFTING HEAVY WEIGHTS.

Intensity

As one of the most important components of an exercise prescription—intensity means how *hard* you work. Age, fitness level and overall health status determine your level of intensity. To prescribe and monitor exercise intensity, various techniques are used. For example, two such methods are heart rate and rating of perceived exertion. These methods offer a guide for monitoring, and therefore controlling the intensity of exercise.

Optimal cardiovascular conditioning occurs when the intensity of exercise maintains a heart rate between 60% to 85% of a maximal heart rate—the target heart rate range. Cardiovascular improvements are *less* with exercise *below* a target rate. Exercising *above* a target range adds little or no improvement to the cardiovascular system, and places you at a greater risk of injury and MVPS symptoms.

Because MVPers often have inappropriate heart-rate responses to physical activity, a target heart-rate range may not be appropriate. To control exercise intensity, therefore, rely on a rating-of-perceived exertion (RPE) scale. The degree of overall effort exerted during exercise is rated on a scale of 1 to 10. A rating of 2 equates with exercise done easily and without strain. A rating of 10 means the exercise is so difficult you can't continue.

RATING OF PERCEIVED EXERTION SCALE

1	Very, very easy
2	Very easy
3	Easy
4	
5	Somewhat hard
6	
7	Hard
8	Very hard
9	
10	Very, very hard

Some MVPers may wish to use a target heart rate (THR) range. Although a maximal graded exercise test gives a more accurate determination, there are other methods of calculating a THR range.

One method is to estimate your target heart rate range. First, subtract your age from 220 to determine your predicted *maximal* heart rate. For example, the age-predicted maximal heart rate for an MVPer of 30 years is 190 bpm—beats per minute. Next, determine your target heart rate *range*. Take 60 percent (.60) to 85 percent (.85) times your *maximal heart rate*. If you are 30, your target heart rate range is 114 to 162 beats per minute.

Another method, Karvonen's method, considers your resting heart rate (RHR) and is more accurate. To obtain RHR—your resting pulse rate—do so immediately before arising, when you are comfortable and rested. Then, enter your RHR into the following formula:

KARVONEN'S FORMULA

RHR = resting heart rate
MHR = maximum heart rate

(MHR − RHR) × .60 + RHR =
                        the lower end of your target heart rate range
(MHR − RHR) × .85 + RHR =
                        the upper end of your target heart rate range

For example, an MVPer of 30 years, with a resting heart rate of 70, age-predicted maximum heart rate (MHR) is 190. [220 − 30 = 190 bpm.] Use these numbers with Karvonen's Formula to establish the target heart rate range at 142 to 172 bpm.

(MHR − RHR) × .60 + RHR(MHR − RHR) × .85 + RHR
(190 − 70) × .60 + 70 = 142(190 − 70) × .85 + 70 = 172

Therefore:

142 bpm (beats per minute) = lower end of target range
172 bpm (beats per minute) = upper end of target range

For exercise to be effective, the workout needs to be intense enough to maintain the heart rate within this range.

Obtaining Your Pulse Rate

(1) Carotid pulse: Place your index and middle finger lightly on your carotid artery. To find this artery locate your Adam's Apple. Next, slide your fingers into the groove next to it.

OR

(2) Radial pulse: Place your index and middle fingers on the thumb side of the inside of your wrist to find your radial pulse.

Count your pulse for 10 seconds. Multiply this number by six. This gives your heart rate per minute.

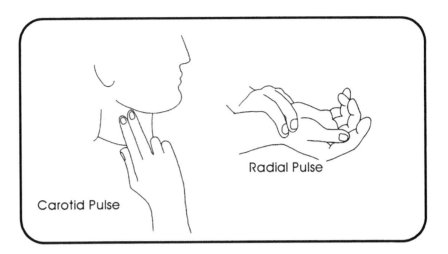

Carotid Pulse

Radial Pulse

When exercising, you should not feel dizzy, fatigued, breathless, or overexerted. Furthermore, you should not experience undue muscle pain or fatigue. One way to gauge your exercise intensity is your ability to converse with a friend. If you are huffing and puffing, barely able to speak, your exercise intensity is too hard. If, however, you can talk comfortably and the work feels somewhat challenging, you are working at the proper intensity. The proper intensity—working hard enough—equals a perceived exertion of *somewhat hard* on the RPE scale.

If the exercise is too difficult, decrease your workload. If the exercise is too easy, increase your workload. Remember: intense, unaccustomed activity often aggravates MVPS symptoms.

Type of Exercise

Any activity that uses large-muscle groups is appropriate if it is rhythmic and aerobic, and is maintained at the proper intensity and duration. Exercise that meets these criteria include walking, bicycling, rowing, jogging, cross-country skiing, aerobic dance, and swimming. *If you presently do not exercise on a regular basis, start with a low-intensity activity such as walking on a level surface.* As your fitness level improves, try other types of more intense activities such as aerobic dance, cross country skiing, or walking uphill.

Find an activity you enjoy. If you dislike biking, don't join a club with only bikes—you won't exercise. Combine types of activities. In addition to adding variety, you tone different muscle groups. Try different types of aerobic activity on different days. Do not assume, however, that because you are conditioned to one type of activity, you will be conditioned for others. Different exercises strengthen different muscles. This is known as training specificity. Unless you do a specific exercise regularly, your muscles may tire and become sore. If, therefore, you begin a new exercise, start slowly.

Types of Aerobic Exercise: Advantages, Disadvantages and Tips

Find one or more of the following that you enjoy, that fits your lifestyle, and that you tolerate. If you have trouble with your knees, ankles, hips, or back, stay with non-weightbearing activities—swimming or bicycling—or with low-impact activities—walking or low-impact aerobics.

Aerobic Dance

For people who like to exercise to music and like to exercise in groups, aerobic dance is perfect. Aerobic exercise combines calisthenics and dance steps with music. Compared with other forms of exercise, aerobic exercise is relatively inexpensive. You can take a class or rent a tape.

Two types of aerobic dance are low-impact and high-impact aerobics. Low-impact requires one foot to always be on the ground. This reduces the stress on joints and, in turn, injury that sometimes occurs with traditional forms of aerobic dance. The intensity of low-impact aerobics varies from low to high, and depends upon the extent of exaggeration of the exercise movement. In other words, the more you move your arms and the higher you lift your legs, the greater the intensity of the workout.

High-impact aerobics involve running and jumping. This increases stress on joints, and the risk of injury. In fact, the forces incurred during high-impact aerobics can exceed three times your body weight. If you have back or joint problems, if you are overweight, or if high-impact aerobics causes pain, then low-impact aerobics is a better choice. If you tolerate and prefer high-impact aerobics, limit this to every other day. This helps decrease the risk of injury.

If you don't exercise regularly, don't start with aerobics. Many MVPers experience undue fatigue when starting an aerobics class. Increase your fitness level first—start a walking program. When you can walk at a brisk pace for a minimum of 20 minutes, sign up for the class.

Before you enroll, make certain the instructor is qualified. Choose one who is certified by a reputable organization, one who is enthusiastic, and one who motivates you to regularly exercise. Find a class that follows appropriate exercise guidelines including warming-up and cooling-down.

Work at you own pace—that's crucial. If the workout feels hard, do not exaggerate your movements—move your arms less, or not at all. Instead of running, march in place. Exercise to a perception of *somewhat hard*. Remember, avoid abrupt postural changes.

Be certain your body positions are correct. This avoids soreness and injury. Keep your feet and knees pointing in the same direction. When running in place or jumping, be sure to roll your feet from your heels to your toes. This helps prevent your calf muscles from getting sore, cramped, or injured. Most important, wear proper, well-fitting shoes. Avoid wearing running shoes. Because of the specificity of foot-impact mechanics, running shoes, along with most other athletic shoes, are not suitable for aerobic dance.

Aerobic Dance Shoes

Look for:
- Impact protection—especially midsole
- Good arch support
- A gradually sloping sole—not the steeper sloping sole found in running shoes
- Adequate toe and heel padding
- Breathable uppers
- Traction that prevents slipping, but doesn't grab the floor
- A sturdy saddle (sides of the shoe) that provides stability for side-to-side motions
- A heel counter—the cup at the back of the shoe that wraps around the heel of the shoe—for lateral stability to the heel area
- Flexibility

Air Bike

Not only does an air bike provide an excellent nonweight-bearing cardiovascular workout, it also tones your arm and leg muscles. Fan blades give the bike its air resistance. The faster you pedal, or the harder you pull, the greater the resistance. You can reach your target heart rate, or a perception of *somewhat hard*, easier with an air bike than with ordinary stationary bikes. Therefore, begin slowly.

Start by warming up at an intensity of *fairly light,* or at less than 1.0 Kilopond. Next, gradually increase the intensity, alternately exercising your arms and legs. Rest your arms every other minute. This allows them to gradually adjust to the exercise. Continue to exercise to a perception of *somewhat hard.* If the exercise feels too intense, pedal slower. If the workload is too easy, pedal faster.

Avoid using *only* your arms, especially if you are deconditioned. Contracting muscles help pump the increased amount of blood needed during exercise. Arm exercise involves a smaller muscle mass than leg exercise. With arm exercise, less help is offered by the contracting muscle mass to pump blood throughout the body. To compensate, your heart rate increases. Therefore, exercise your arms and legs together—your heart rate won't increase as rapidly. Remember, cool down the same way you warmed-up.

In addition to upright bikes, air bikes are available in fully and semirecumbent positions. Recumbent bikes have a bucket seat, have pedals that are more in front—rather than directly underneath—and are more comfortable for those with low back pain.

Arm Ergometer

An arm ergometer is like a bike for your arms. While you are seated or standing, your arms spin a crank at varying speed and intensity. Arm ergometry is a good cardiovascular workout and it also tones your arms and shoulders. Most people, however, do not have the arm strength to maintain the intensity and duration required for an aerobic exercise session. Furthermore, arm work can cause an abrupt increase in heart rate.

Despite its difficulties, it is useful to add three to five minutes of arm ergometry to your workout. This helps strengthen your upper body and adds variety to your workout. For those who want to use only an arm ergometer, alternate rest periods with spinning the crank until you feel fatigued.

Although you can sit while cranking the arm ergometer, it is best to stand and move your legs. Standing and moving counters gravitational forces, avoids blood pooling in your legs, and promotes recirculation of blood. This is particularly important for MVPers with symptoms of dizziness or lightheadedness.

To exercise, begin by turning the intensity knob to zero resistance. Set the timer for two or three minutes. Position yourself at a comfortable proximity to the arm crank. Begin turning it at a speed of 50 revolutions per minute. Gradually increase the speed. If you feel any discomfort, slow down the cranking speed.

Bicycle Ergometer

Bicycle ergometers—stationary bicycles—are non-weightbearing, tone leg and buttock muscles and give you a cardiovascular workout. If you are deconditioned, a stationary bike is a good first choice. You can exercise at low-to-moderate intensities. A disadvantage, however, is that your legs will fatigue before you achieve your target heart rate. To reduce leg fatigue, decrease the resistance and increase pedal speed. As your cardiovascular fitness improves, move to a higher intensity exercise that you can perform without being limited by leg fatigue. If you have access to both a standard stationary bicycle and an air bike, progress to an air bike after a few weeks of using the stationary bicycle. For further comfort and lower back support, use a recumbent bike.

To help pass the time while riding a stationary bike, work out with a friend, exercise to music, or exercise watching television. You might want to buy an inexpensive magazine stand, attach it to your bicycle, and read while you ride.

The stationary bike seat must be properly adjusted. To do this, stand next to the bike and adjust the seat so it's approximately at hip level. Next, climb on the bicycle and put the balls of your feet on the pedals. When each pedal reaches its lowest point in the cycle, your leg should be slightly bent—almost straight—you should not strain to reach the pedal.

To adjust the tension, first remove all tension from the bicycle wheel by adjusting the appropriate knob. Next, begin pedaling. You can't accurately adjust the tension till you pedal at your workout speed. Pedal at 50–60 revolutions per minute. Follow the guidelines in this chapter for details about duration, intensity, frequency, progression, and proper warmup and cool down.

Warm up with little to no intensity—about 0 to 20 Watts per 50–60 rpm (revolutions per minute). Next, continue to pedal at 50 to 60 rpm. Gradually increase the tension till the work feels *somewhat hard.* After your workout, decrease the tension and cool down.

Bicycling Outside

Outdoor bicycling is easy to learn and gives you the opportunity to sightsee. It is non-weightbearing, can be performed at a low-to-high intensity, and requires only a sturdy bicycle and comfortable clothing. To be safe, especially if riding near automobile traffic, invest in a bicycle helmet.

Prices for bicycles vary from a standard, inexpensive bike to an expensive, deluxe racer. Before you buy, compare prices. Check a cyclist's magazines or *Consumer Reports.* Ask a reputable bicycle dealer or experienced cyclists for advice.

Dress for comfort and protection from the weather. Wear shoes with heavy soles, and wool or cotton socks. Tuck shoe laces in, and secure pants cuffs so they don't get caught in the chain. If you plan on biking regularly, invest in a pair of shoes made specifically for biking.

Although rain or snow may prevent you from cycling outside, you can buy rollers or indoor trainers for indoor riding. Cycling on rollers or indoor trainers mimics your outdoor-bicycle workout better than riding a stationary bike.

Proper frame size and bicycle seat, as well as proper handlebar adjustment, are important for comfort and safety. As you stand in bare feet, the bicycle frame size should be nine to ten inches less than your inseam measurement. The inseam measurement is the distance between your crotch and the floor. Because of variations such as tire size, this formula doesn't always hold true. Therefore, always straddle the bike you intend to buy. Then, barefoot, with both feet flat on the floor, be certain the top tube of the frame is 3/4" to 1" below your crotch.

Sit on the bike. Then, adjust the seat's height.

Next, center your heel on a pedal at its lowest point in the cycle.

With your pelvis level on the seat, fully extend your legs.

To ride, pedal on your toes and slightly bend your knees. Your leg should be fully extended while your pelvis is level on the seat. For information about any other adjustments, ask a salesperson, or refer to the handbook.

To begin your workout, ride on a flat surface and use low gear. Keep the intensity *fairly light* for five to ten minutes. Pedal continuously at a comfortable pace. Usually, the pedal speed is faster than that of a stationary bike—about 70–90 rpm on an outdoor bicycle versus 50–60 rpm on a bicycle ergometer. Increase the intensity to *somewhat hard.* To do this, increase the gear, pedal faster, or ride up a hill. Remember, you want to ride continuously for 30 to 40 minutes. Coasting does not count. Cool down the same way you warmed up.

Cross-Country Skiing

Cross-country skiing is an all-around exercise—it combines hiking and skiing. It is low impact and uses both arms and legs rhythmically and continuously, making it an excellent source of cardiovascular conditioning. Cross-country skiing also tones all of the major muscles and muscle groups.

While good weather conditions are needed to ski outside, there are cross-country ski simulators for indoor use. If you buy one, make certain the skis glide smoothly, and there is an intensity adjustment for both arms and legs.

Cross-country skiing requires a lot of cardiovascular endurance, muscular strength, and coordination—*it is not for people starting to get into shape.* The intensity of cross-country skiing is such that it is difficult for most people to endure for a complete exercise session. Therefore, if you are beginning an exercise program, first get into shape. Start with lower-intensity activities such as walking or biking. Then, gradually add a few minutes of cross country ski-simulator activity to your workout. Alternate intervals of three-to-five minute rest periods as you exercise on the ski simulator.

Gradually increase your workout time. Use the cross-country ski simulator for the entire workout, or alternate the ski simulator with periods of a lower-intensity exercise.

If the ski simulator has a support pad, adjust it to hip level. Press lightly against the pad when cross-country skiing, but keep your weight on your feet—not on the pad. Move your legs back and forth until you get your balance. Keep your knees slightly bent and use a comfortable stride. With the toes of one foot, push one ski back, and keep your other foot flat as it glides forward. Once you feel comfortable using only your legs, add your arms. Alternate each arm forward with the opposite leg. If your right arm is forward, then your left leg is forward. Swing your arms like pendulums—extend your arm until your elbow is straight. Cross-country skiing takes coordination and lots of patience to master.

Jogging

Jogging is inexpensive, lets you enjoy the outdoors, and offers excellent cardiovascular conditioning. Jogging, however, is associated with a higher risk of injury than other non-weightbearing or low-impact activities. It places the stress of three times your body weight on your joints, your back, and rest of your body. If you are overweight or have trouble with your knees, ankles, hips or back, don't jog. Swimming—a non-weightbearing activity, or walking—a low-impact exercise—is preferable.

If you prefer to jog and are able, do so *no more* than *every other day*. This reduces your risk of injury. If you want to exercise daily, perform a non-weightbearing or low-impact activity on alternate days.

Before you start, choose a good running shoe. Make sure there is at least 1/2 to 3/4 of an inch between your toes and the front of the shoe. Chose one with sturdy arch support and a durable sole. Be certain the sole is a good shock absorber. To minimize up-and-down or side-to-side heel movement, select a shoe with a firm, well-fitting heel counter—a cup at the back of the shoe that wraps around the heel for reinforcement.

For those beginning to exercise, start with a walking program. When you can walk briskly for a half hour, try a combination of walking and jogging. Do this for about twenty minutes. For example, start with repeated intervals of walking two minutes, then walking and jogging thirty seconds. Gradually *increase* the length of the jogging intervals, and *decrease* the length of the walking intervals. Do this till you can continuously jog for 20–30 minutes. Remember to warm up before, and to cool down after. For example, walk or slowly jog for five to ten minutes both before and after your jog.

Develop an appropriate running style to maximize jogging efficiency and comfort, as well as to prevent injuries and soreness. Make certain you land on your heel, and roll off of the ball of your foot. Breathe normally through your mouth and nose;

relax your arms and shoulders. Ask an experienced runner, athletic trainer, or other sports-medicine professional to check your running style and correct serious errors.

Rowing

Rowing, an excellent source of cardiovascular exercise, tones most of the major muscle groups with little stress on your joints. Rowing, however is not a good choice if you have back or knee problems. Because rowing is a more intense exercise and difficult to perform for an entire workout, use the rower for only a few minutes as part of your workout.

If you are beginning an exercise program, do not start with rowing. First, perform less intense cardiovascular actives to develop cardiovascular fitness.

Properly use the rowing machine to maximize cardiovascular conditioning and to decrease your risk of injury and back strain. As you pull back with your arms, push back with your legs. Initially, keep your hands facing downward—overhanded. At times, row underhanded—hands facing upward—to strengthen your biceps. Do not extend your legs to the point that your knees lock.

Next, slide forward. Repeat this cycle rhythmically. Keep your back straight and perpendicular to the floor throughout the rowing cycle. If you feel any discomfort in your back, or other part of your body, make sure that your rowing technique is correct. If you still experience discomfort, then discontinue rowing as a component of your fitness program.

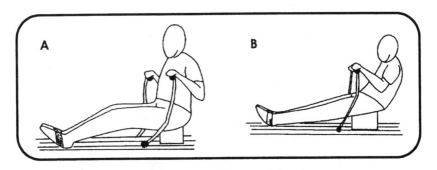

A. Proper Rowing Technique   B. Improper Rowing Technique

To begin, warm up for three to five minutes; adjust the resistance to the lowest level; and row at a speed that feels *fairly light.* For your first few sessions, the warmup period adequately accustoms your body to this piece of equipment. Later on, increase the intensity of your workout until it feels *somewhat hard.* To do this, increase the resistance, or increase the speed. In general, a good pace is 20 to 25 strokes per minute. When you finish, cool down for five minutes at the same intensity with which you warmed up.

Stair Machine

A stair machine provides a very good low-impact cardiovascular workout. It works all of the major muscles in the lower part of your body: muscles in your legs, hips, and buttocks. If, however, you have weak ankles, knees, or quadriceps, a stair machine may not be your best choice.

It is best to first strengthen weakened ankles, knees, or quads with other lower-intensity aerobic activity.

Intensity on a stair machine is a function of step height, stepping speed, and the resistance you work against. To start, first adjust the resistance to a low level. Next, adjust the step height to 6 or 8 inches. Increase and decrease the intensity of your workout by the stepping speed. Follow the previously described guidelines for warming up, working out, and cooling down.

If you experience discomfort in your knees, ankles, or elsewhere while using a stair machine, make sure the step height is not adjusted too high. If this does not correct the problem, then stop using stair machines.

Swimming

Swimming is an excellent source of cardiovascular conditioning, is non-weightbearing, and can tone all of the major muscle groups in your body. Because your body weight is supported by water, swimming is less stressful on your joints than most activities. Therefore, the risk of injuries in swimming versus high-impact activities is much lower.

The energy cost of swimming is about four times that of running an equal distance. While energy is needed for your arms and legs to propel you through the water, energy must also be expended to keep you afloat. The drag of the water also provides excellent resistance that improves muscular strength and endurance.

As compared with someone who does the same amount of work and achieves the same cardiovascular benefits with land sports, the swimmer's heart rate will be lower. In fact, studies show that when someone swims, her maximum heart rate averages 13 beats per minute less than it would on land. Therefore, if you use a target heart rate to monitor the intensity of exercise, subtract 13 from your actual or your age-predicted maximum heart rate before using it in Karvonen's equation.

To warm up, swim slowly for 5 to 10 minutes at an intensity that feels *fairly light*. Then, swim more briskly for 20 to 30 minutes at an intensity that feels *somewhat hard*. To finish, swim slowly for 5 to 10 minutes to cool down. As part of your warmup or cool down, you may hold on to the edge of the pool and gently kick your legs.

Walking

Walking requires no special skill and, except for a good pair of walking shoes, no special equipment. It is an excellent activity for people starting to get into shape, as well as for experienced athletes. Furthermore, while walking puts the stress of *one and one-quarter times* your weight on your joints and back, jogging puts approximately *three times* your weight on your body.

A good pair of walking shoes maximizes safety, comfort, and enjoyment. Look for shoes with more flexibility than a running shoe—ones that have extra shock protection at the heel, which is the focus of impact. Choose ones that have good arch support to absorb shock that would otherwise be transmitted to your body. Be sure the shoe is durable, with a stiff toe box, a breathable upper (top of the shoe), and with plenty of space between your toes and the front of the shoe.

As you get into shape, increase the intensity of your workout. Increase your walking pace; swing your arms more; walk uphill; or add light wrist weights—two pounds or less per arm.

Walking Outside

Walking outside is enjoyable and beneficial. It allows you to explore the outdoors while you become physically fit. Too, you may socialize and make new friends through noncompetitive walking clubs—such as Volksmarching clubs—and organization-sponsored walks for charity. To walk with a friend or with a group also motivates you to continue your fitness program.

If the weather is bad, continue to walk at a mall or at a fitness center* for a good reason. Suppose you are now in shape physically from first walking on a flat surface. It's time to increase the *intensity* of your exercise program. Why? After a few weeks of conditioning, your cardiovascular system gets stronger. Now, it takes a higher degree of intensity to both increase your heart rate and to feel that the exercise is *somewhat hard.*

How can you do this? Increase your walking pace to a fast, comfortable pace. If the exercise still doesn't feel *somewhat hard,* wear one-or-two-pound wrist weights and swing your arms more. Should this strain your shoulders, don't use the weights. Furthermore, don't add ankle weights. They place added stress on your joints and back. Rather, to increase intensity, walk up some hills.

Walking in the Mall

Walking in a local shopping mall offers a free, often convenient alternative to walking outside. It has the advantage of offering shelter from rain, snow, and extremes of temperature. Many shopping malls keep hallways open both before the shops open, and after they close. Mall-walkers' clubs offer group support, camaraderie, and instruction. Contact you local chapter of the American Heart Association for helpful information. Determine which local malls welcome walkers; what is the mileage of the various local malls; and which local malls support walking organizations.

Again, remember to increase the *intensity* of your walk. Increase your walking speed. If necessary, wear one-to-two pound wrist weights. Then, vigorously swing your arms.

Walking on a Treadmill

Walking on a treadmill offers a more controlled workout intensity. By increasing its grade or slant, you achieve the same intensity as a jog. But, unlike a jog, you add no stress to your joints. Walking on a treadmill does not tone any muscles in

---

*Some fitness centers let you pay on a single-session basis.

your arms. To get a complete workout, add arm work such as using light, free weights or using an air bike.

Proper use of a treadmill is necessary for maximum safety and to achieve cardiovascular benefits. First, before you turn on the treadmill put *one foot on either side of the conveyer belt.* Turn on the power and the conveyor belt. Then, adjust the speed. If you are out of shape and don't know what speed to start with, begin at 1.5 mph. Tap one foot on the belt to get a feel for the speed of the treadmill. Begin to walk on the treadmill. Take comfortable strides. Keep your hips under your shoulders; keep your arms and shoulders relaxed; and keep your body near the front of the treadmill. Walk heel to toe. Experiment till you find a speed that feels *fairly light* and warm up for five minutes. Gradually work up to an intensity that feels *somewhat hard.*

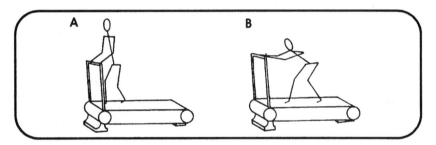

A. Correct Position: Walk erectly near front of belt, hand(s) resting on handrail or at your side.
B. Incorrect position: Walking bent over hanging onto handrail for support.

Gradually work up to the fastest speed with which you're comfortable. Once this no longer feels *somewhat hard,* gradually increase the grade or slant of the treadmill by 2% to 3%. Walk for at least two minutes at each increase in the grade. During your last 5–10 minutes, gradually decrease both the grade and speed of the treadmill. Don't get off till the treadmill is flat and the belt hardly moves.

Finally, turn off the treadmill, step off, but keep moving. Continue your cool down. Walk slowly for a few minutes. You may feel slightly dizzy when you step off a treadmill because your body develops a forward momentum without actually moving forward. When you stop, your body retains some of this momentum. Some MVPers experience more dizziness. If you stop to catch your balance, the problem worsens. Blood has already pooled in the legs. By standing still, gravitational forces further cause blood to pool in the legs. This lowers blood pressure in the upper body and causes more dizziness. Dizziness decreases once you cool down and walk around for a few minutes.

Frequency of Exercise

Regular exercise is an important component of a fitness program. For MVPS symptom control, schedule exercise at least three times a week on alternate days. Although daily exercise doesn't harm the cardiovascular system, it can put excess stress on your joints. Therefore, limit high-impact activities — jogging or jumping—to alternate days.

Duration and Progression of Training

Your present level of fitness determines the initial duration of your exercise session. While some MVPers start with 30 minutes of exercise, others barely make ten. Either way, ten minutes of exercise is better than zero minutes of exercise.

If you begin an aerobic exercise program, start with 10 to 20 minutes of exercise. Add two to five minutes each session until you reach 30 to 45 minutes. This time *does not* include warmup and cool down.

Overall improvement depends upon your initial level of fitness—the lower your fitness, the greater the improvement. Adjust your exercise prescription as improvements in fitness and conditioning occur. Once you achieve cardiovascular conditioning—maintain it.

SIGNS OF IMPROVEMENT

Signs that regular aerobic exercise is increasing the efficiency of your cardiorespiratory system include:

- A lower resting heart rate
- A lower heart rate while doing the same amount of work
- A post-exercise heart rate that more quickly than before approaches your normal resting heart rate
- An increase in your endurance during exercise and normal daily activities
- A decrease in the intensity and frequency of MVPS symptoms

Exercise Prescription: Muscular Fitness

Aerobic exercise is the most important type of exercise for someone with MVPS. But, do *add* exercises that develop muscular tone, strength, and endurance. Take special care to properly perform these exercises, and thereby avoid aggravating MVPS symptoms.

Many women worry that lifting weights develops large, bulging muscles. In fact, women get much less hypertrophy—increase in muscle size—than men do. Change in muscle size is mediated by the hormone testosterone, which is present in much lower levels in women.

PRINCIPLES TO CONSIDER WHEN DEVELOPING A WEIGHT TRAINING PROGRAM

- Overload
- Progressive resistance
- Specificity
- Arrangement of exercises
- Frequency
- Duration
- Safety

Principles of Strength Training

Consider the following principles as you develop a strength-training program.

(1) *Overload Principle*: To strengthen a muscle, it needs to work against more resistance or lift more weight than usual.

(2) *Progressive Resistance Principle:* To reach your desired level of strength and endurance, gradually increase the amount of resistance applied. To maintain this level of muscular strength and endurance, continue to lift the same amount of weight.

(3) *Specificity Principle*: The development of muscular fitness is specific to the muscle group exercised, the type of contraction, and the intensity of exercise. In other words, weight-training programs should exercise muscles you actually use in

sports or in everyday activities. They should also mimic both the movement patterns and intensities involved.

(4) *Principle of Arrangement of Exercises*: To achieve maximum benefit from a training session, exercise your larger muscles before your smaller ones. Smaller muscles aid larger muscles. If you first exercise the smaller muscles, they will fatigue. Consequently, this limits the amount of weight the larger muscles and muscle groups can lift. Similarly, arrange training programs so no two successive exercises involve the same muscle or muscle group.

EXERCISE MUSCLE GROUPS IN THE FOLLOWING ORDER	
First	Upper legs and hips
Second	Chest and upper arms
Third	Back and posterior legs
Fourth	Lower legs and ankles
Fifth	Shoulders and posterior upper arms
Sixth	Abdomen
Seventh	Anterior upper arms

Type of Strength Training Exercise

Strength training exercises include isometric, isotonic, and isokinetic. For MVPers, the most appropriate is *isotonic* exercise. Isotonic exercises include sit-ups, crunches, using a weight station, and lifting free weights—hand weights or barbells.

Intensity

(*Caution:* If you note an increase in MVPS symptoms, try lighter weights. Then, if you still can't tolerate weight lifting, stop. Do other types of exercise.)

To lift weights, start with ones that are easy to lift, and ones you can comfortably lift at least eight times. Women: try two to five pounds. Men: try five to ten pounds. To increase muscular endurance, gradually increase the repetitions—the number of times a weight is lifted without a rest. Add one or two repetitions per exercise session till you lift the weight 15 times. Then, you can increase the weight.

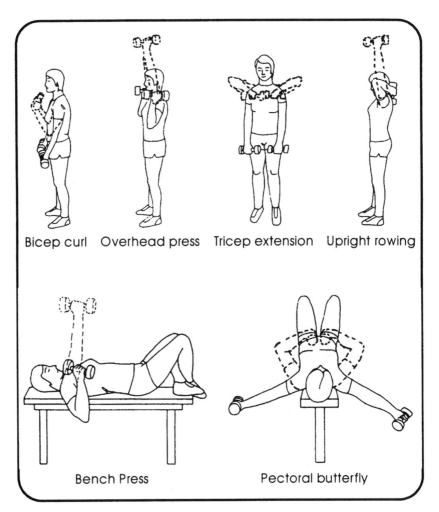

Bicep curl   Overhead press   Tricep extension   Upright rowing

Bench Press   Pectoral butterfly

ISOTONIC CONTRACTIONS USING FREE WEIGHTS

How much weight you lift depends on your tolerance of the weight, your fitness level, and the types of your daily activities. An exercise physiologist, sports medicine physician, or physical therapist can help determine your weight limit. In general, female MVPers can gradually work up to 20 to 30 pounds without an increase in symptoms. Many male MVPers tolerate even higher weights. Remember, start out with light weights, and increase weights *gradually*. Decrease the weight if you note an increase in symptoms.

Frequency

Studies show that muscles respond best after a day of rest. Why? Part of the muscle-strengthening process involves partially tearing down muscle tissue and rebuilding stronger tissue. Therefore, perform muscular resistance exercises only two to three, nonconsecutive days per week.

Duration

The duration equals the amount of time it takes to perform the prescribed number of repetitions and sets—groups of repetitions that alternate with rest periods. Duration is more important with cardiovascular exercise than with weight-resistance exercise.

Additional How To's

Always consult your physician before starting a weight-training program.

Warm up before you lift weights. First, stretch the muscles that you will use. Next, perform the same movements that you will do while lifting weights. Do this with either a light weight or no weight for a few repetitions.

Never hold your breath when exercising. As you lift a weight, *slowly exhale* to prevent a spike in blood pressure. Slowly perform this initial movement to the count of two. Let the weight down slowly to the count of four. The movement of letting the weight down produces most of the strength-building benefits. Therefore, do this slowly.

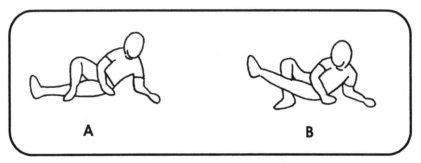

A. PROPER ADDUCTOR LIFT (INNER THIGH LIFT)
B. IMPROPER ADDUCTOR LIFT (INNER THIGH LIFT)

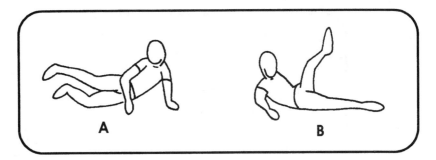

A. PROPER ADDUCTOR LIFT (OUTER THIGH LIFT)
B. IMPROPER ADDUCTOR LIFT (OUTER THIGH LIFT)

Crunches versus Sit-ups

During the first few degrees of a sit-up you use your abdominal muscles. Then, you use the muscles in your back, which may lead to back strain. A better way to strengthen your abdominal muscles, is with a *crunch*—a modified sit up. To do a crunch:

1. Lie on the floor with knees bent, feet flat, and arms crossed over your chest.

2. As you lift your upper body by contracting your abdominal muscles, leave your lower back flat on the floor. Exhale as you lift up.

3. Lift no more than a 30- to 45-degree angle.

4. To a *slow* count of four, inhale as you lower your upper body to the floor.

To prevent neck strain, only lift with your abdominal muscles. Let your head come up with the rest of your body.

To help prevent lower back strain, always keep your legs bent. Do not hook your feet under a bar or piece of furniture—otherwise, your hips and legs do most of the work. To work the sides of the abdominal area more effectively, add a slight twist to some of your crunches. Move each shoulder towards an opposite leg.

Start with five to ten crunches. Add one or two crunches per session till you work up to 20 to 30. If you tolerate them, you can perform up to 45 crunches. Divide these into three sets of 15 repetitions with brief periods of rest in between. Doing more will not be helpful. To make them more of a challenge, perform the crunches more slowly.

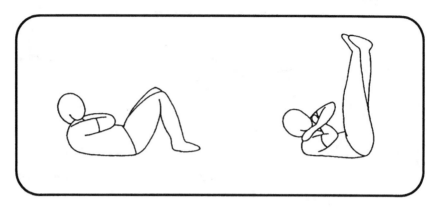

A. Proper Crunch   B. Crunch Variation

Weight Station

A weight station is a piece of equipment with which you can work all of the major muscles and muscle groups in your body. Consult a sports medicine professional for guidelines on the proper use of this equipment.

General Exercise Tips

When should you eat and drink relative to exercise?

Never exercise immediately after you have eaten. Allow at least one hour after a light snack and two hours after a regular meal.

Be sure to replace the extra fluids lost during exercise. Drink plenty of water before, during, and after exercise. During heavy exercise, replace fluids with eight ounces of water every 15 minutes. Also, avoid drinking caffeine prior to exercise. This may have an adverse effect on blood flow to the heart muscle during exercise.

Be sure to replace the extra fluids lost during exercise. Drink plenty of water before, during, and after exercise. During heavy exercise, replace fluids with six to eight ounces of water every 15 minutes.

TABLE 6-1

- **Twenty-four hours before exercise**
  Consume a nutritionally balanced diet
  Drink adequate fluids.

- **Two hours before exercise**
  Drink 500 ml (about 17 oz) fluid

- **During exercise**
  Drink cool (15° to 20°C), palatable fluids at a rate of 4–8 oz every 15 to 20 min

- **For exercise less than 1 hour**
  Water is adequate for hydration and rehydration

- **For exercise longer than 1 hour**
  Fluids, including 4% to 8% carbohydrate and/or electrolyte, may improve hydration or performance

- **After exercise**
  Drink 16 to 20 oz fluid for every pound lost during exercise. Including sodium may promote more rapid recovery, but it is not necessary as long as sodium is sufficiently available from food.

SOURCE: The American College of Sports Medicine.

Unless you have high blood pressure, or your physician recommends that you reduce your sodium intake, use salt freely. The electrolytes in your food generally replace those lost during exercise, except during prolonged, intense events such as marathons. Unless the event is over 90 minutes long, only water needs to be consumed during exercise.

What should you wear?

Wear proper athletic shoes along with breathable, cotton socks both to reduce the risk of blisters and to absorb moisture. Wear loose-fitting, comfortable clothing. Choose cotton or wool fabrics because they allow skin to breathe. There are also several breathable, man-made fabrics such as Lycra, Gore-Tex Waterproof, polypropylene, and Coolmax. Wear layers to avoid the effects of wind and cold. Consult with sales representatives at reputable sporting goods stores, or sports medicine professionals, or refer to related literature for further information.

When should you either avoid or lessen the intensity of exercise?

Avoid exercise if you don't feel well. Cold, fever, infection, diarrhea, or vomiting increase the metabolic demands of your body and increase your heart rate. Similarly, if you are tired, hot, have a slight cold or allergies, decrease the intensity and duration of your workout.

Avoid exercising in extremely warm (above 90 degrees and 80% humidity) or cold (below 32 degrees) weather. Decrease the intensity if you exercise in temperatures between 80 and 89 degrees. If you stay within the guidelines for RPE (Rating of Perceived Exertion scale), you automatically adhere to these temperature and illness guidelines.

What if you experience symptoms during exercise?

If you experience symptoms, such as palpitations, excessive fatigue, chest pain, or discomfort, excessive shortness of breath, or any unusual symptom, decrease your level of intensity. If the symptoms persist, cool down and stop exercising.

What if you want to buy some exercise equipment?

Before you buy any exercise equipment, be sure you'll use it. Often it soon becomes a dust collector. Many people become motivated by taking a fitness class, by joining a fitness club, or by exercising with a friend.

Before you invest, experiment. Either use a friend's equipment or find a fitness facility that will let you try out different pieces of equipment. See what your body tolerates, and what you enjoy.

Once you decide upon a piece of equipment, try to get one that is used or in good repair. But, before you buy, try it out to make sure the equipment is sturdy, in good repair, and easy to operate. For tips about advantages and disadvantages of specific types of exercise, exercise equipment, and how to use it, refer to the section **Types of Exercise**.

What about performing activities in high altitude?

Physical performance is reduced at high altitudes and may be particularly bothersome for MVPers who enjoy hiking or skiing in the mountains. Subjective feelings of fatigue may be more pronounced than at sea level. Also, the heart may beat faster and the heartbeat may feel more forceful.

To avoid this uncomfortable sensation, maintain a slower tempo. Perform the activity at a reduced intensity for less time. Don't push beyond a perception of *somewhat hard.* It takes longer at higher altitudes than at sea level to recover from intense activity. Remember to drink plenty of fluids prior to, during, and after your trip.

What about participating in athletic sports activities?

Sports activities include everything from auto racing to water polo, and individual clinical situations vary. *Participating in athletic sports, therefore, should be discussed with your physician.* In general, your physician considers the degree of mitral regurgitation—back flow of blood flow into the left atrium, presence and type of arrhythmias, size of the heart chambers, your clinical history, your symptoms, and type of sports activity.

Myths about Exercise

No pain, no gain: Pain is a warning sign that you need to back off. You risk injury or an increase in symptoms if you continue. Warm up; cool down properly; don't intensely work out, and follow the guidelines discussed. You shouldn't have pain.

I can spot-reduce fat from certain areas of my body: You can't spot-reduce fat. You lose fat by burning more calories than you consume. Where you lose fat depends on your sex and your heredity. While exercises like sit-ups or crunches strengthen and tone muscles, they don't spot-reduce fat.

Exercise turns fat into muscle: Although aerobic exercise burns fat, and both weight resistance and aerobic exercise improve muscle tone, they don't turn fat to muscle. For example, consider the big, muscular football player who becomes fat. He's accustomed to consuming enough calories to support an active, young body. As he gets older, he no longer remains physically active. His muscles atrophy—weaken and shrink in size—from lack of exercise. To top this off, he still eats as usual. Because he consumes more calories than he burns, he gets fat.

I am too old to start exercising: You are never too old to start exercising. Thousands of people in their 60's, 70's, and 80's begin exercise programs. It's inspiring to consider the tremendous gains in fitness they achieve.

I don't have enough energy to exercise: This is all the more reason to exercise. Within a few weeks exercise increases energy levels. Start slowly; be patient; and enjoy the results.

I don't have enough time to exercise: Make time. You'll find that regular cardiovascular exercise increases alertness, promotes self confidence, and increases energy levels. You may find, therefore, you become more efficient and accomplish more tasks with less fatigue. Ask yourself, "Am I worth giving up only three hours a week to better condition myself?"

Housework, golf, bowling, and chasing after small children is enough exercise: These activities can be tiring. They can improve flexibility. They can improve muscular strength. But they don't meet the criteria for aerobic exercise. They don't provide benefits that cardiovascular exercises do.

Exercise will always increase your appetite: If you are normal weight and begin an exercise program, your appetite may increase slightly to compensate for the extra calories that you burn. If you are overweight and begin an exercise program, the exercise may actually help your body regulate your appetite.

Walking a mile quickly will burn more calories than walking a mile slowly. Regardless of how quickly or how slowly you walk a mile, you burn about the same number of calories. Of course, if you walk a mile quickly, you burn the calories faster—you burn more calories per hour—not per mile.

Passive exercise helps burn calories and helps you get stronger without the work: Passive exercise, such as riding on an electrically operated bicycle, may improve flexibility. It doesn't give you aerobic or muscle-toning exercise. To strengthen muscles, you have to work against a resistance. Remember, whichever one does the work—the machine or you—gets the benefits.

References

American College of Sports Medicine. 2000. Guidelines for Exercise Testing and Prescription. 6th ed. Lea & Febiger. Philadelphia.

Astrand, P.-O. & K. Rodahl. 2003. Textbook of work Physiology. 4th ed. McGraw-Hill Book Company. New York.

Baumgartner, R., C. Chumlea & A. Roche. 1990. Bioelectric impedance for body composition. *In* Exercise and Sport Sciences Reviews. K. Pandolf & J. Holloszy, Eds.: 193–224. Williams & Wilkins. Baltimore.

Boudoulas, H. & C. Wooley. 1988. Mitral valve prolapse: Childhood, pregnancy, athletics, and aviation. *In* Mitral Valve Prolapse and the Mitral Valve Prolapse Syndrome. H. Boudoudas & C. Wooley, Eds.: 609–631. Futura Publishers. Mount Kisco, New York.

Borg, G. 1970. Perceived exertion as an indicator of somatic stress. *Scandinavian Journal of Rehabilitative Medicine* **2-3:** 92–98.

Convertino, V., L. Armstrong, E. Coyle, G. Mack, M. Sawka, L.C.J. Senay *et al.* 1996. American College of Sports Medicine position stand: Exercise and fluid replacement. *Medicine and Science in Sports and Exercise* **28**(1): i–vii.

Fletcher, C. 1984. The Complete Walker III. Alfred A. Knopf, Inc. New York.

Fox, Edward L., Timothy E. Kirby & Ann Roberts Fox. 1987. Bases of Fitness. Macmillan. New York.

Francis, L.L., P.R. Francis & K. Welshons-Smith. 1985. Aerobic dance injuries: a survey of instructors. *In* The Physician and Sports Medicine, 13(2). McGraw-Hill, Inc.

Froelicher, V. 1987. Exercise and the Heart: Clinical Concepts. 2nd ed. Year Book Publishers, Inc. Chicago.

Fontana, M., C. Wooley, R. Leighton & R. Lewis. 1975. Postural changes in left ventricular and mitral valvular dynamics in the systolic click-late systolic murmur syndrome. *Circulation* **51:** 165–173.

Graves, J., M. Pollock, S. Montain, A. Jackson & J. O'Keefe. 1987. The effect of hand-held weights on the physiological responses to walking exercise. *Medicine and Science in Sports and Exercise* **19**(3): 260–265.

Graves, J., A. Martin, L. Miltenberger & M. Pollock. 1988. Physiological responses to walking with hand weights, wrist weights, and ankle weights. *Medicine and Science in Sports and Exercise* **20**(3): 265–271.

Guyton, A.C. 1986. Textbook of Medical Physiology, 7th ed. W.B. Saunders Co. Philadelphia.

Health Letter Associates. 1988, December. The best all-around exercise. *University of California, Berkeley Wellness Letter* **5**(3): 6.

Health Letter Associates. 1987, March. Swimming to a different beat. *University of California, Berkeley Wellness Letter* **3**(6): 7.

Health Letter Associates. 1990, May. What if you did 5,000 sit-ups a month? *University of California, Berkeley Wellness Letter* **6**(8): 6.

Holland, H.J., J.J. Hoffmann, W. Vincent, M. Mayers & A. Caston. 1990. Treadmill vs. steptreadmill ergometry. *The Physician and Sportsmedicine* **18**(1): 79–85.

Iskandrian, A.S. 1988. Exercise left ventricular performance in patients with mitral valve prolapse. *Urban & Vogel* **13**(4): 243–248. Herz, Philadelphia.

Jackson, A.S. & M.L. Pollock. 1978. Generalized equations for predicting body density of men. *British Journal of Nutrition* **40:** 497–507.

Jackson, A.S., M.L. Pollock & A. Ward. 1980. Generalized equations for predicting body density of women. *Medicine in Science, Sports & Exercise* **12:** 175–182.

Koszuta, Laurie Einstein. 1987. Can fitness be found at the top of the stairs? *The Physician and Sportsmedicine* **15**(2): 165–169.

Lamb, D. 1984. Physiology of Exercise: Responses and Adaptations. Macmillan. New York.

Loften, M., R. Boileau, B. Massey & T. Lohman. 1988. Effect of arm training on central and peripheral circulatory function. *Medicine and Science in Sports and Exercise* **20**(2): 136–141.

Maresh, C, & B. Noble. 1984. Utilization of perceived exertion ratings during exercise testing and training. *In* Cardiac Rehabilitation: Exercise Testing and Prescription, L.K. Hall, Ed.: 155–173. Spectrum Publications, Inc.

Marino, J., L. May & H. Bennett. 1981. John Marino's Bicycling Book. J.P. Tarcher, Inc. Los Angeles.

Maron, B. & J. Mitchell. 1994. 26th Bethesda Conference: Recommendations for determining eligibility for competition in athletes with cardiovascular abnormalities. *Journal of the American College of Cardiology* **24:** 845–899.

Monahan, T. 1988. Perceived exertion: an old exercise tool finds new applications. *The Physician and Sportsmedicine* **16**: 174–179.

Namdar, M., P. Koepfli, R. Grathwohl, P. Siegrist, M. Klainguti, T. Schepis, *et al.* 2006. Caffeine decreases exercise-induced myocardial flow reserve. *Journal of the American College of Cardiology* **47:** 405–410

Nieman, D. 1986. The Sports Medicine Fitness Course. Bull Publishing Co. Palo Alto, CA.

Pollock, M., & D. Mason, D. (1986). Heart Disease and Rehabilitation, 2nd ed. John Wiley & Sons. New York.

President's Council on Physical Fitness and Sports. 1971. Physical Fitness Research Digest, Series 1, No. 1. Washington, DC.

Rosiello, R., D. Mahler & J. Ward. 1987. Cardiovascular responses to rowing. *Medicine and Science in Sports and Exercise* **19**(3): 239–245.

Scordo, K. 1991. Effects of aerobic exercise in symptomatic women with mitral valve prolapse. *American Journal of Cardiology* **67**: 863–868.

Scordo, K. 1996. Taking Control: Living with the Mitral Valve Prolapse Syndrome, 2nd ed. Kardinal Publishing. Cincinnati.

Skinner, J., R. Hutsler, V. Bergsteinova & E. Buskirk. 1973. The validity and reliability of a rating scale of perceived exertion. *Medicine and Science in Sports* **5**(2): 94–96.

Wilmoth, S. 1986. Leading Aerobic Dance-Exercise. Human Kinetics Publishers, Inc. Champaign, IL.

7

Anxiety, Panic Attacks, and MVPS

"I feel crazy."
"I'm going to die."
"I'm going to faint."
"I feel so out of control."
"My whole body is tingling."
"Everyone will notice how foolish I am."
"I know I'm going to have a heart attack."
"I can't go in that store ... that's where I had my last attack."

Sound familiar? For those with panic attacks, these are common thoughts. Research studies confirm that many MVPers do have anxiety and panic attacks. The connection between the two, however, remains unclear. A heightened autonomic nervous system may be partly responsible.

Before you begin this chapter, see how much you already know. Take the following quiz. Check either true or false.

QUIZ

1. To feel anxiety means I fail to cope.
   True _____ False _____

2. If my heart palpitates and my hands tingle, a fatal heart attack follows.
   True _____ False _____

3. Panic attacks come out of the blue.
   True _____ False _____

4. I can do nothing about panic attacks.
   True _____ False _____

All of the above statements are false. Now, read on.

Remember, there's *no cure* for MVP, but you *can learn* to peacefully co-exist with it. Don't turn over your life to chronic heath conditions such as MVPS, arthritis, hypertension, or dia-betes. If you do, expect to feel like a *cork bobbing in the ocean* — always waiting for the next big wave, shark, or typhoon. A help-less, out-of-control feeling leads to depression, anxiety, pho-bias, or panic attacks. Right now make it a goal to take charge of your life. How?

Become knowledgeable. Knowledge *is* power. Carefully read, re-read and *study* this chapter because panic attacks *don't come out of the blue.* How then, might *you* trigger these attacks? How can you avoid them?

Anxiety

Webster defines anxiety as a state of being uneasy, apprehen-sive, or worried about what *might* happen—a concern about some *possible* future event. Anxiety is a normal living experi-ence: physically, emotionally, socially, spiritually, and psycho-logically.

The word anxiety is sometimes misconstrued. Anxiety, for example, is the psychological siren of the human organism. Remember your first date, your wedding day, the birth of your first child? How did you feel? Did your heart pound? Were you faint, dizzy, or weak? Would it be fair to say that you felt anx-ious? Yes, of course.

Throughout life, anxiety normally occurs at various develop-mental transition points. Children learn to crawl and walk because they're frustrated *and* anxious. They want the shiny red ball across the room. As their hearts pound, and their limbs tremble, they move under their own power for the first time. Thus, they overcome their anxiety and grow. In moderation, anxiety encourages growth. In excess, anxiety paralyzes and sometimes causes panic attacks.

What produces anxiety in one person doesn't necessarily pro-duce anxiety in another. For example: Some people fear flying. Others fear driving. Some fear open spaces. Others fear con-fined areas.

Research demonstrates that anxiety and panic are controlled and governed by an individual's *perception.* How you perceive something influences your emotions—the way you think and the way you feel. If you perceive MVPS symptoms as cata-strophic, you *encourage* a panic attack. Alter your *perception,* and you control it. *You* are the only one who is in charge of your panic attacks.

Anatomy of Panic Attacks

What kinds of feelings characterize panic attacks?

In the absence of any *external* threats, brief episodes of intense fear occur and surface as physical symptoms. They often inflict terror and a fear of losing control. Symptoms may last several seconds or for several minutes. Anyone who has experienced an attack characterizes it as frightening and most uncomfortable. In fact, you sometimes momentarily think, "I'm losing my mind." Panic attacks resemble fight-or-flight responses. For example: Suppose you walk in Central Park in New York at midnight and suddenly hear a strange sound. Bursts of catecholamines—adrenaline-like substances—activate and circulate throughout your system. Now, you shake; you perspire. Your heart pounds; your muscles tense; your breathing accelerates. You prepare to flee or to fight.

In much the same way, this area of the brain that controls the fight-or-flight response stimulates and sets off panic attacks. But, now this alarm—this danger response—occurs even though there's no real danger.

A panic attack often occurs following any form of severe stress caused, for example, by divorce, illness, job change, work overload, serious accident, or loss of a family member. (Also, excessive consumption of caffeine or use of stimulant medications may trigger panic attacks.) How you respond to these stressful life events may be influenced by your level of anxiety sensitivity—excessively heightened vigilance. For example, an individual with high levels of anxiety sensitivity who has a fear of palpitations may be at a greater risk for panic disorder. Often, the higher the level of anxiety sensitivity, the greater the likelihood of stress-induced physical symptoms of anxiety or fear that ultimately end in a full-blown panic attack.

With recurring panic attacks, it is not uncommon for you to *anticipate* another attack. This behavior—fear of having another panic attack—is called *anticipatory anxiety*. Afflicted persons become apprehensive and often begin to avoid any events and circumstances likely to trigger attacks. For example, if you had your first or worst anxiety attack while driving, anticipatory anxiety may keep you from driving again. As more attacks occur in different settings, the person's activities may become increasingly limited. Family, social, and professional activities become severely disrupted. The person may become agoraphobic.*

Agoraphobia affects approximately one-third of all people with panic disorder. They fear being in any place or situation where escape might be difficult, or where help is unavailable in the event of a panic attack. Commonly, people with agoraphobia fear crowds, standing in line, entering shopping malls, and riding in cars or in public transportation. Often, their comfort zone includes only their home or immediate neighborhood. At times, they may travel if accompanied by a friend. Even when they are in their comfort zone, they may continue to have panic attacks.

PANIC ATTACK SYMPTOMS

During a panic attack, any or all of the following symptoms occur:

- Chest pain or other chest discomfort
- Chills or hot flashes
- Choking sensation
- Derealization (feeling unreal) or depersonalization (feeling detached from self)
- Feeling dizzy, lightheaded, faint ,or unsteady
- Fear of dying
- Fears of loss of control or becoming insane
- Heart pounding, racing, or skipping beats
- Nausea or other abdominal discomfort
- Numbness or tingling
- Sweating
- Shortness of breath or smothering sensation
- Trembling

Source: *Diagnostic and Statistical Manual of Mental Disorders*, 4th edition (DSM-IV). 1994. The American Psychiatric Association, Washington, DC.

Agora is Greek for marketplace. Agoraphobia literally means fear of the market place—a fear of crowds of people assembled there.

Perceptions

Research indicates that panic attacks may result from the catastrophic misinterpretation of certain bodily sensations. This is illustrated below.

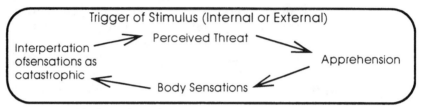

Source: Clark, D. (1986).

To apply this illustration, think of *internal trigger stimuli* as palpitations, dizziness, or chest pain, and of *external stimuli* as flying, driving, shopping in supermarkets. Any stimulus perceived as a threat causes you to become apprehensive. For example, you may say, "I hope I don't have a panic attack while I'm driving." Soon, your heart pounds; your chest hurts; and you become short of breath. Each bodily sensation intensifies with apprehension. Each sensation becomes catastrophic. You're convinced that because you have a heart problem and chest pains, you're going to die.

In Chapter 1 you learned that your autonomic nervous system automatically becomes stimulated by *perceived* threats. Your body normally responds and causes you to perspire, to feel breathless and dizzy, or to note pounding heartbeats. If these normal physical responses are misinterpreted as catastrophic, the panic cycle feeds on itself and perpetuates.

Studies show that *panic attacks are triggered by a physical sensation* such as palpitations. In turn, the physical sensation increases both awareness and an anxiety level that intensifies the physical responses of the autonomic nervous system. This is interpreted as catastrophic, and the threat is intensified. Finally, anxiety escalates to panic level and sends the autonomic nervous system into overdrive. To try and stop a panic attack at this point is similar to putting your car in reverse while driving 70 miles an hour.

"OUT OF THE BLUE?"

An exchange between an MVP program participant, Laura, and the seminar leader follows.

Laura: "My last panic attack occurred at home as I sat at my computer. Nothing happened to cause it. The attack literally came out of the blue. What do you mean it didn't?"

Seminar leader: "Let's explore the time period before the attack."

Laura: "It wasn't a good week. My husband was out of town. I always get edgy when he's away. *I'm afraid something will happen.* It never has, but it could. I'm responsible for three little children—you never know what can happen."

She further recalled, "I ate a large meal before I began to work. Eating a full meal frequently causes palpitations. I remember I had palpitations when I first began to work at my computer."

Now, Laura began to place the panic attack into its proper context. As she explored the time period immediately *before* the attack, she realized her palpitations were more intense than usual. She believed she was going to die. As the palpitations intensified, she became even more anxious than usual.

Because the physical symptom is perceived as very intense, there's an increased risk of misinterpreting it as catastrophic. When Laura put the situation into perspective, it became apparent that her physical symptom—palpitations—was misinterpreted catastrophically. Faced with a perceived threat, she had no choice but to have a panic attack.

As you saw, the time and place to act on an impending attack is *before* it happens—*before* you interpret harmless, normal physical signs (palpitations, tingling, dizziness) as *catastrophic.* Prevent your autonomic nervous system from going into overdrive.

If you don't like *how* you feel about yourself, about your life, and about your symptoms, *change how you think.* It's the key to taking control of anxiety and panic attacks. How? Try cognitive therapy.

Cognitive Behavioral Therapy (CBT)

Cognition includes all forms of knowing: perceiving, judging, conceiving, reasoning, and remembering. According to cognitive behavioral therapy, abnormalities of behavior and mood result from abnormal thinking. Cognitive therapy, therefore, gives priority to thinking and not to feelings. It is a helpful tool to use on your own.

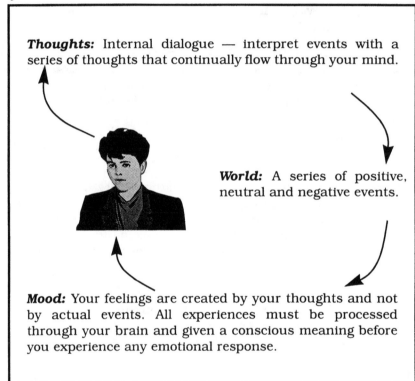

Thoughts: Internal dialogue — interpret events with a series of thoughts that continually flow through your mind.

World: A series of positive, neutral and negative events.

Mood: Your feelings are created by your thoughts and not by actual events. All experiences must be processed through your brain and given a conscious meaning before you experience any emotional response.

Source: Burns, D. (1980).

Guiding Principles of Cognitive Therapy

Principle 1—Automatic Thoughts. Moods and feelings are influenced in the here-and-now by automatic thoughts and cognitions. These automatic thoughts create a stream of ideas that repeatedly and insistently intrude upon our conscious awareness.

Examples of problematic automatic thoughts associated with MVPS: "I have MVPS; something is wrong with my heart. If my heart goes, my body follows." Whenever this MVPer has palpitations his thought process *will* interpret palpitations as catastrophic.

Principle 2—Thought Traps or Cognitive Distortions: Pessimistic thoughts that cause depression and anxiety frequently are unrealistic, illogical, and distorted. A common denominator in thought distortions is *negativity*. When nothing is good and nowhere is safe, chronic depression and high-level anxiety ensue. *Reality doesn't cause* unhealthy feelings such as depression or anxiety. Rather, negative thoughts about reality contribute.

Ten forms of cognitive distortions, or twisted thinking, that create negative emotions include:†

1. *All-or-Nothing Thinking*: You see everything as black and white with no gray areas. You're a total failure if one aspect of your life is less than perfect. EXAMPLE: If your boss makes a minor correction on your report, you know he will fire you. You're incompetent.

2. *Overgeneralization:* You set up a self-fulfilling prophecy of defeat based on one negative event. EXAMPLES: The alarm failed to go off this morning. You're sure the car won't start. You'll be late for work. Your boss will hate your presentation. By tomorrow morning, you'll be a bag lady.

3. *Mental Filter:* You focus on a single negative detail and create a dark reality. EXAMPLE: After you receive many compliments on your presentation, someone recommends using blue instead of black ink. You leave the meeting depressed.

4. *Discounting the Positive:* You insist your positive qualities or accomplishments don't count. EXAMPLE: Your sister says you look like a knockout in your dress. You politely tell her what she says doesn't count—she's family.

5. *Jumping to Conclusions:* In the absence of accurate information, you believe the worst.

    (a) *Mind reading*: You assume everyone dislikes you.

    (b) *Fortune-telling:* You predict that everything will turn out badly.

EXAMPLE: Although your friend was on the second level of the mall and you were on the first, surely she intentionally ignored you. She didn't wave hello. She will never talk to you again.

---

†Burns, D. 1980. Feeling Good: The New Mood Therapy; and Burns, D. 1993. Ten Days to Self Esteem. See references for further information.

6. *Catastrophizing or Minimizing:* You discount the positive and accentuate the negative. EXAMPLE: Because your friend complains for hours about how she had to change part of her presentation, you empathize. Even though the company accepted *your* proposal you say how *bad* it is.

7. *Emotional Reasoning:* You believe that your worst fears and feelings are reality. EXAMPLE: You receive a call. The boss wants to see you. Since this could only mean he wants to fire you, you suffer a panic attack on the elevator en route to his office.

8. Should *Statements.* You criticize yourself or others with *shoulds.*

Shoulds usually indicate two seemingly conflicting sets of needs. Failure to choose between the two and accept the consequences causes discomfort. EXAMPLE: I should visit my parents every week. Mothers should meet all the needs of all members of their family. Men should never show weakness. I should never feel anxious. I should never get angry. I should never have palpitations if my heart is truly OK.

9. *Labeling:* You make yourself the sum total of what you do; you attach value to yourself *based only on what you do.* EXAMPLE: Instead of saying, "I forgot to make the appointment—I made a mistake," you tell yourself, "I'm a loser—I can't do anything right."

10. *Personalization:* You see yourself as the *cause* of every negative event with which you come in contact. EXAMPLE: Your husband is angry and short with you. You know *you* caused it.

As you see, to feel *bad* about yourself comes from distorted thought patterns. Distorted thoughts won't let you feel *good* about yourself. What can you do? Replace negative, unrealistic thoughts with positive, realistic thoughts. Yes, you *can* change the way you feel.

Positive reinforcement and good feelings about yourself are the sustenance that feeds a stable and secure sense of self. MVPers who possess a stable and secure self usually operate at a relatively low anxiety level. Furthermore, the less daily anxiety you experience, the less likely you are to perceive MVPS symptoms as life threatening and to panic.

Principle 3—Believing in Incorrect Assumptions about Oneself and One's Self-esteem. Attaching your self-esteem, or sense of well-being to the success of a project, to the response from another, or to the presence or absence of a mistake, makes feeling good impossible. Faulty assumptions cause fear, anxiety, and panic.

Examples of faulty assumptions: Because you haven't had palpitations in a week, you'll never have them again. If MVPS is harmless, you should never have any symptoms. Believe your worth as a human being depends on what you do.

In each of these situations, you assume a cause-and-effect relationship between non-related items. Example: MVPS is not curable. Expect occasional symptoms. Don't base your sense of well-being on never having any symptoms. You'll set yourself up for anxiety and panic attacks.

Furthermore, the belief that self-worth depends on one's achievements leads to a roller-coaster ride through life. One's self-worth and self-esteem come from inside. You'll note that it is called *self*-esteem, and not *the-other-person-gives-it-to-you*-esteem. It's a constant sense of knowing who you are, why you are the way you are, and what you believe you're capable of doing in any situation. If you're only as good as your project, you hand over responsibility for how you feel about yourself to other people, that is, to a committee or to anyone who approves your project. These people don't take responsibility for *your* self-esteem. Instead, they concern themselves with only *their own* self-esteem. Therefore, only *you* can assume responsibility and determine how you feel about yourself.

Although feedback is important, place it in the context of your entire social, physical, spiritual, psychological, and intellectual being. You *are* more than the sum of all the tasks you've done. To believe otherwise leads to chronic anxiety. Then, everything you do has the potential to make you feel terrible about yourself. How much of that can any one person take without becoming anxious, depressed, and panicky?

Goals of Cognitive Therapy

To take control, strive to achieve the following goals:
1. Pinpoint automatic thoughts, thought traps, and silent assumptions that trigger and perpetuate anxiety or panic-attack cycles.
2. Identify the distortions or cognitive errors.
3. Substitute more realistic, self-enhancing thoughts that reduce painful feelings.
4. Replace self-defeating, silent assumptions with more reasonable belief systems.

If you now believe: My heart pounds; I have chest pain; I have MVPS; I'm having a heart attack, change your thinking. Say to yourself, "I've had this before; this is not new to me. I didn't die before, and I'm *not* going to die now."

Continue to perceive your palpitations as catastrophic, and you choose to have a panic attack. Don't perceive them as catastrophic, and choose to avert an attack. Remember, *you can recreate the perception you created.*

Start your own personal cognitive therapy now. Think about your last attack. What happened in your life the day before, the hour before the attack? Complete the *Thought Analysis Sheet* (Burns, 1993). Fill in the spaces in whatever order you remember.

At the top of the sheet, briefly describe the situation that led to your physical response. In the first column, list any physical symptoms you felt: palpitations, chest pain, numbness, or shortness of breath. Next, record your emotional response and any cognitive distortion. In the last column, write a rational response to your thoughts.

The critical step is the positive or rational response. *Be open and honest with yourself.* Thus, you'll begin to challenge your automatic thoughts, to identify your thought traps, and to discover your anxiety-producing assumptions. Be surprised by the results; but, remember this is a process. Start with hindsight, and realize you lost control just *after the attack.* Now, realize what you did *while it went on* but couldn't stop it. This helps you identify situations that place you at risk of an attack, such as flying, driving, eating, being alone, or during the middle of the night. Although you may still have another attack, you'll know what's happening to you. As you continue to use this process, you'll feel symptoms—tingling, palpitations, chest pain, feelings of unreality—but you'll recognize them. Although you're scared, you'll know they are normal, but not fatal.

Remember **ANXIETY IS NOT TERMINAL.** Anxiety, and its physical manifestations, are normal occurrences. Catastrophic misinterpretations of the body's *normal* response to *normal* anxiety cause panic attacks. Although cognitive therapy is *not* a substitute for medicine or for psychotherapy, it is a useful tool. It provides a structure for altering the incidence of panic attacks. Start now. Use the work sheet. Soon you'll be able to mentally complete the sheet.

Examples:

Situation: *I have to drive to the supermarket where I had my first anxiety attack.*

THOUGHT ANALYSIS SHEET

PHYSICAL SYMPTOM	COGNITIVE DISTORTION	POSITIVE THOUGHT
Heart pounding	I'm going to die (Emotional reasoning)	I've had heart pounding before. I can do pursed-lip breathing and feel better.

Situation: *My husband is out of town. I worry that something might happen to me and my children will be alone.*

THOUGHT ANALYSIS SHEET

PHYSICAL SYMPTOM	COGNITIVE DISTORTION	POSITIVE THOUGHT
Chest pain	I'm going to have a heart attack. (Catastrophizing) (Emotional reasoning)	Nothing has ever happened that I couldn't handle when he was out of town. I don't like being alone, but I can manage. Actually, chest pains are part of MVPS, and my fear makes them worse.

Situation: *The boss wants to see me now. I decide to take the stairs to his office.*

THOUGHT ANALYSIS SHEET

PHYSICAL SYMPTOM	COGNITIVE DISTORTION	POSITIVE THOUGHT
Short of breath Dizziness Heart pounding	I'm going to be fired. He hates me. My heartbeat is going to kill me. (Emotional reasoning) (Catastrophizing) (Emotional reasoning)	I don't know what the boss wants. My fear makes my MVPS symptoms worse. If I breathe deeply and slow my pace down, I'll be fine.

Situation: _____

_____

THOUGHT ANALYSIS SHEET

Physical Symptom	Cognitive Distortion	Positive Thought

Medications

For completeness, medications often prescribed for the treatment of panic attacks are discussed below. The intent of this section is to provide information, *not* to recommend one drug over another, nor suggest you start taking medication. For many, symptoms are managed without medication. Some people, however, may temporarily need or want medication to get over the hump. Together with your health care provider discuss the use of medication, its purpose, its effectiveness, and its accompanying guidelines.

Commonly used medications known to be effective to treat panic attacks include: (1) SSRIs (selective serotonin reuptake inhibitors); (2) tricyclic antidepressants; (3) benzodiazepines; and (4) MAO (monoamine oxidase) inhibitors. The pharmacological actions of the drugs are complex and beyond the scope of this chapter, and thus a brief overview of these four classes of drugs is provided.

There are currently six SSRIs available in the U.S.: citalopram (Celexa), escitalopram (Lexapro), fluoxetine (Prozac), fluvoxamine (Luvox), paroxetine (Paxil) and sertraline (Zoloft). All of these agents are effective, although not all of them have been FDA-approved for use in panic disorder. SSRIs reduce the intensity and frequency of panic attacks, reduce anticipatory anxiety, and treat associated depression. Some forms of depression, however, have a major anxiety component that can induce anxiety symptoms. Therefore, treatment of depression can decrease anxiety and decrease the risk of panic attacks. These drugs work by affecting serotonin, a naturally occurring neurotransmitter that functions as the body's calmative substance. These medications increase the availability of serotonin in the body, and therapy helps to prevent panic attacks. The main side effects of SSRIs are headaches, irritability, nausea and other gastrointestinal complaints, insomnia, sexual dysfunctions, increased anxiety, drowsiness, and tremor. To avoid the possibility of withdrawal or discontinuation symptoms, unless otherwise instructed, do not abruptly discontinue these drugs. Instead, taper the dose over several weeks.

Tricyclic antidepressants (TCAs)—clomipramine (Anafranil), imipramine (Tofranil), and nortriptyline (Aventyl)—also help to reduce the intensity and frequency of panic attacks, and may prevent anticipatory anxiety. Common side effects include dry mouth and constipation. To alleviate dry mouth, chew sugar-free gum or hard candy. To minimize constipation, increase your water intake to at least eight glasses per day. If water doesn't help, drink prune juice, increase your fiber intake, or use a mild laxative. Notify your health-care provider should you experience sweating, extreme nervousness, blurred vision, or flushing of the face.

Benzodiazepines—alprazolam (Xanax), clonazepam (Klonopin), diazepam (Valium), and lorazepam (Ativan)]—also reduce the intensity and frequency of panic attacks, anticipatory anxiety, and may lead to a reduction in phobic avoidance. Alprazolam is the most extensively studied of this group of medications. Side effects are primarily sedation, fatigue, ataxia, slurred speech, memory impairment, and weakness. Because of a tendency for dependence, these drugs should only be used for the short term. A gradual taper of no more than a 10% reduction in daily dose per week, and tapering over at least 2-4 months is recommended. Be advised that withdrawal symptoms might occur throughout the tapering period, especially toward the last half of the period.

A group of antidepressants known as MAO inhibitors are also used to treat panic attacks—phenelzine (Nardil) and tranylcypromine (Parnate). Side effects include sleep disturbance, weight gain, and sexual dysfunction. When you take MAO

FOODS TO AVOID WITH MAO INHIBITORS

- Beer and wine, particularly Chianti
- Cheese, except cottage and cream cheese
- Smoked or pickled fish, especially herring
- Beef or chicken liver
- Summer sausage—dry
- Fava or broad bean pods—Italian green beans
- Yeast vitamin supplements—brewer's yeast
- Ripe fresh banana
- Ripe avocado
- Sour cream
- Soy sauce
- Yogurt
- Yeast breads
- Raisins
- Figs
- Meat tenderizers
- Chocolate
- Caffeine-containing beverages

inhibitors, *closely monitor your diet.* Foods that contain high amounts of tyramine can interact with MAO inhibitors and cause serious side effects such as a sharp, dangerous rise in blood pressure.

In addition to dietary recommendations, avoid over-the-counter medications that contain vasopressor substances—ephedrine or phenylpropanolamine such as Contac or Dristan. Be certain your physician gives you information about any dietary and medication restrictions.

Antidepressants take at least 14 days to reach full effect. When you become stabilized at a dose, you should notice a decrease in the frequency of panic attacks. It may take several months, so don't stop the medicine because you feel better and haven't had a panic attack. Your body needs to finally take over and do what the medicine did. Work with your physician to gradually decrease the medicine over a period of time. If panic attacks return during withdrawal, one of two things might be happening. First, you may have a chemical imbalance. This may require continued treatment with medication. Second, perhaps

A twenty-eight-year-old woman cancelled two appointments with the MVP Program. Each time, enroute to the center, she suffered panic attacks. The third time her husband drove, and she had no problem.

It was three months after her daughter's birth that panic attacks began. She endured a difficult pregnancy—was on bed rest the last three months—and then delivered a baby who became colicky. Needless to say, the new mother's panic attacks increased in intensity and in frequency. Furthermore, with her husband's transfer, they now lived in a city 200 miles from the only home she ever knew.

At the MVP Program, we began a family history. Although she knew little about MVPS, she remembered her father's taking medication for nerves. Her sister, an aerobics instructor, seemed to be high strung, but kept it under control with exercise. She then asked if a lack of exercise may have played a role in *her* own panic attacks. Ever since high school and until pregnancy, she ran 25 miles a week.

I said, "YES. Exercise produces endorphins that are involved in the synthesis of serotonin. Serotonin is the neurotransmitter involved in mental alertness and systemic calming. Through exercise you previously compensated for an apparent familial chemical imbalance."

Together, we developed a plan that involved diet, exercise, and thought analysis. She agreed to follow the plan for three months. *Unless* she experienced a decrease in frequency and intensity of her panic attacks, she would return. Only then would we discuss medication to help her bring a degree of control and mastery into her life. For two years now, I have not seen her.

you depended solely upon the medicine and did little to help yourself.

Minor tranquilizers or anti-anxiety agents such as alprazolam (Xanax) or lorezepam (Ativan) are used either to stop or prevent an attack when conditions seem conducive. These agents relax you and help you to think better. Less anxious, you'll be less inclined to catastrophically interpret something. If you're in the throes of an attack, Xanax may help blunt the symptoms.

Anti-anxiety agents are addictive, and in time you'll require higher doses to do the job. If you took several a day and *every day* for many months, work with your physician to gradually decrease the dosage and discontinue the medication. Remember, medication *does not cure* the problem. You must continue to work at helping yourself.

Frequently Asked Questions about Anxiety and Panic Attacks

1. What is the difference between anxiety, generalized anxiety disorder, and panic disorder?

Anxiety is normal; generalized anxiety disorder (GAD) is not. Anxiety means perceiving something as threatening, such as taking a driver's test. Excessive anxiety and worry about events or activities may signal GAD. For those with GAD, the anxiety symptoms of apprehension, worry, irritability, difficulty in concentration, insomnia and somatic (bodily) complaints are present more days than not for at least 6 months.

A panic attack is a discrete period of intense apprehension, fearfulness, or terror, often associated with feelings of impending doom, that usually lasts for a short period of time (e.g., 10 minutes). Panic disorder occurs when there are recurrent, unpredictable attacks followed by at least one month of persistent concern about having another panic attack, worry about the possible implications or consequences of the panic attacks, or a significant behavioral change related to the attacks.‡ Panic disorder does not include panic attacks that are attributed to physiological effects of a general medical condition, a substance or another mental disorder. Panic disorder may be associated with the development of agoraphobia—anxiety about or avoidance of certain situations from which escape or help is not possible should a panic attack occur.

------

‡American Psychiatric Association. 1994. Diagnostic and Statistical Manual of Mental Disorders, 4th ed. (DSM-IV). American Psychiatric Association. Washington, D.C.

2. Are there any factors that make individuals more susceptible to panic disorder?

As previously mentioned, not everyone responds to stressful life events with panic attacks. What makes some people more vulnerable to panic disorders than others is a complex phenomenon, not completely understood and beyond the scope of this book. Genetic make-up may be one factor. Research studies of families and twins demonstrate that there is a genetic propensity to develop panic disorders. Whether this genetic contribution is general or specific is not certain. Either way, genes seem to play a role in some component of the vulnerability for panic attacks.

Research also shows that people who were raised in an environment that afforded them control or a sense of mastery over their environment, including their emotional lives, are less likely to develop panic disorder than those who did not have this control. Thus, having an enhanced sense of mastery and control may immunize a person against later anxiety. Conversely, multiple experiences with uncontrollable stressors may enhance vulnerability to anxiety. Although controversial, it is thought that *early* stressful life events such as parental death, separation, or divorce, may enhance vulnerability to development of panic disorder and agoraphobia later on in life.

3. I've had MVP for years, and panic attacks that start and stop. How come?

Panic attacks often come and go during changes in your life. Here is one theory:

In the growing fetus, the nervous system and the heart develop simultaneously. If one develops defectively, so may the other. The result might be but a *hair trigger* on your fight-or-flight response. Compared with most people, an MVPer's autonomic nervous system can respond quicker, and with greater intensity. When this sensitive nervous system is subjected to a series of stressors that occur within a short period of time, a panic attack can occur. This is called the *kindling effect*. The faulty nervous system may predispose you to the development of symptoms. With the right amount of stressors, in the right amount of time, a panic attack ensues. You may, however, never develop symptoms till your life situation challenges.

Stressors are *kindling* for the development of panic attacks. For example: Are you starting a new job, moving away from home, getting a divorce, fighting with your neighbors, raising a family, and working full time? These are typical major stressors that can cause panic. But it doesn't need to be a major stressor. Instead, an assortment of minor stressors may cause panic attacks. For example, the kids are sick. The baby sitter quit. Your car broke down, and your mother wants to go shopping today. Whatever raises your daily anxiety level beyond baseline increases your risk of having a panic attack, as well as increasing the intensity and frequency of MVPS symptoms. The cycle goes on.

4. What do I do when I'm having an attack? How do I cope with a panic attack?

When you have a panic attack, the goal is to keep safe while you ride it out. In its early stages, walk around and concentrate on deep breathing. This may blunt or calm symptoms. Physical activity gives panic impulses along your nervous system some competition. If you have someone you can talk to, call that person. If a tranquilizer has been prescribed for you, take it. The medicine helps you to relax and lessen the intensity of your symptoms. As you relax and consider these symptoms to be normal, your autonomic nervous system switches from fight-or-flight to a steady, controlled state.

If all attempts fail and you seriously feel that you are going to die, go to an emergency room. You and your well-being are worth it.

Remember, the time to act on a panic attack is *before* it happens. Stopping a Ferrari at full throttle is difficult. As soon as possible after a panic attack use the Thought-Analysis Sheet. Identify which perceptions induced an attack. Replace misinformation with correct information. You control your perceptions. You control panic attacks.

5. Is it possible to awaken at night with an anxiety attack?

Yes. Through dreams we take care of any issues, concerns, and feelings that we failed to address during the day. Combined with even low levels of stressful, depressing, and anxiety-producing events, a panic attack can occur during sleep. Thus, when we fail to remember the dream that perhaps precipitated an attack, we entertain weird thoughts. For example: "I must be dying because I can't find any reason *why* I'm having a panic attack." Then, when sleep becomes a problem, the baseline-anxiety level escalates. Hence, the cycle intensifies and perpetuates.

As one approach to solving this problem, place a pen and a note pad beside your bed. Say to yourself before retiring, "I *will* remember my dreams tonight." As soon as you awaken, write *whatever* you remember about the dream. From these bits and pieces plus an analysis of you pre-sleep anxiety level, you may learn what caused a panic attack.

6. Is anger related to panic attacks?

Yes. If you are angry, your life may not be going the way you wish. That spells stress. Stress can be acted out or expressed through a weakened body part as, for example, in migraines, ulcers, colitis, spastic colon, and back pain. MVPS symptoms sometimes "act out" stress in a similar fashion. Anger and associated stress can cause an increase in the severity and frequency of symptoms such as palpitations and chest pain. The more intense the symptom pattern, the greater is the likelihood of a catastrophic interpretation and risk of a panic attack. Yes, panic attacks and anger are closely related.

7. Does cognitive therapy really work?

Yes, it does. Cognitive therapy gets you off *automatic pilot*—responding to the symptoms of the panic attack as if you're only along for the ride. Cognitive therapy prepares you to become your own master. You recognize symptoms that evoke panic attacks, learn how to control them, and, in turn, learn how to prevent them in the future.

Said one MVPer "I really let this thing get the best of me. I couldn't even go to the grocery store for fear I'd have a panic attack. Now, I *don't think* I'm about to die with palpitations. Instead, I talk to the palpitations and say, `I know you're there, but I'm busy. Now, let's get over it.' People think I'm crazy, but this works well for me."

8. Are there any other ways to cope with anxiety and panic attacks in addition to using cognitive therapy?

Yes. Learn ways to relax and to keep your anxiety level below threshold. Participate in a cardiovascular-exercise program. Exercise helps *siphon off any charge*. Once anxiety approaches a livable level, you're more inclined to risk uncovering your sources of anxiety.

Relaxation provides a key to self mastery. As you work off frustrations and insecurities through exercise, you put yourself in a positive frame of mind, prepared to uncover and to treat any *sources* of anxiety. Consult a trained therapist to learn about biofeedback—through the use of relaxation tapes.

Become knowledgeable about diet. For example, did you know that carbohydrates play a major role in either preventing or decreasing the intensity of panic attacks? Processing of carbohydrates in the body boosts the availability of tryptophan. Tryptophan—an amino acid involved in the synthesis of serotonin—is the neurotransmitter that helps us control mood, feel calm, concentrated, focused, relaxed, and content.

Unfortunately, because we often eat carbohydrates with protein or fat we *decrease* the availability of tryptophan.

Carbohydrates are an effective anxiety-reducing agent when eaten alone. Recommended servings include: 2 oz. of oyster crackers, 16 animal crackers, 1 plain bagel, 2.5 oz. of pretzels, and 1-1/2 cups of Alpha Bits. Allow 30 minutes to work. Eaten in moderation prior to a high-risk event (driving a car, going to the supermarket, a visit from your mother-in-law), carbohydrates can be an effective, nonpharmaceutical, chemical intervention to reduce anxiety. This intervention is within *your control*—no prescription, no authorization needed.

Remember to avoid foods that create stress. These include caffeine, fried foods, junk foods, and sugar. Also, if you enjoy herbal teas, try catnip, hops, passion flower, chamomile, and valerian root. These have a calming effect.

9. When should I seek help from a therapist?

If, after three months of regular exercise, a modified diet, and use of thought analysis sheets, there is no decrease in either the frequency or intensity of your panic attacks, its time to seek help. Something else is happening. Unless effectively treated, depression, chemical imbalance, or both cause symptoms to persist. Depression or chemical imbalance or both cause symptoms to persist. Interview prospective therapists, as you would new employees. Learn what they know about MVPS Do they use the cognitive approach in the treatment of panic attacks? What is their position on the use of medication to bring panic attacks under control? Then, choose a therapist with an advanced degree—a master's or doctorate—who is associated with a physician. This therapist can work with you on two levels.

On level one, is the use of medication to stabilize your nervous system. Because medication is self-administered, it helps you build a sense of mastery over the panic attacks.

On level two, both your and the therapist address the possible *source* of your depression. Once identified, together, you lay the groundwork for the next step—prevention. Say to yourself, "Although I am responsible for my depression, I also have the willpower to *get* myself out and the willpower to keep myself out." In therapy, *knowledge is power*. Make sure that the therapist you choose *agrees*.

10. My sister and I both have MVPS. I have panic attacks. She doesn't. Why?

Not every person with MVPS even knows that he or she has it. Furthermore, *not everyone* with MVPS has panic attacks. The best explanation of these realities lies in the examination of one's "internal climate."

Everyone operates with a degree of anxiety known as a *baseline*-anxiety level (see diagram). Each person has a panic threshold: the amount of anxiety generated to cause a panic attack. Our baseline-anxiety level fluctuates according to how well we manage ourselves, and how we perceive stresses that come our way. Given enough stressors over a short period of time together with poor stress management, such as thought traps and automatic thoughts, we *can* reach the panic level, and a panic attack ensues.

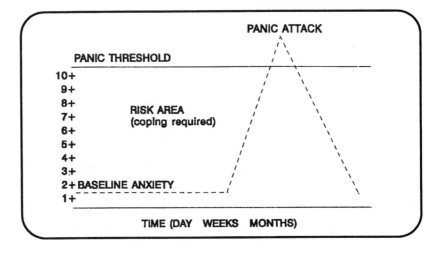

11. How do I deal with friends and family?

The answer is twofold: accept responsibility for the manner in which you *react* to MVPS; *within reason* enlighten friends and family members concerning its symptoms. Explain how they come and go, and why they sometimes become problematical.

Too, no one but *you* can improve your condition. Parents, spouses, children and friends do *not* have the responsibility to make your condition better. To expect others' lives to revolve around *you* invites rejection. If you believe, "If only they would do, say, or be ... I wouldn't have panic attacks," you may feel unloved, depressed, and anxious. Your relationships will be fraught with conflict, blame, and distance. The result is more MVPS symptoms.

To expect others to shoulder responsibility they're unable to do keeps you from gaining mastery over a condition that is *your* responsibility. Once you accept the responsibility for your panic attacks, you allow family and friends to fulfill their role as a support system. They too need information to understand changes you make in relationships. Although friends and family may not appreciate limit-setting and boundary changes, given the proper information, they may be more tolerant. Keep in mind that it's never easy to accept whatever we don't understand.

Summary

You are not alone. Many other MVPers suffer from anxiety and panic attacks. From this book you know that anxiety is a normal human response to a perceived threat. You also know that a panic attack starts when a normal physical reaction to a perceived threat is catastrophically interpreted. Keep in mind that *you are in control* of what is perceived as a threat.

Use cognitive therapy as a tool for you to identify any perceptions, faulty assumptions, and thought distortions that contribute to the intensity and frequency of your panic attacks.

Next, *correct* your faulty assumptions, and get rid of all perceptual and thought distortions. Be determined; begin right now. *Take control* over your anxiety and panic attacks. And, don't forget: *What you think determines how you feel. To like the way you feel, change the way you think.* The choice is YOURS.

References

American Psychiatric Association. 1994. Diagnostic and Statistical Manual of Mental Disorders (DSM-IV), 4th ed. American Psychiatric Association. Washington, D.C.

American Psychiatric Association. 1998. Practice guideline for the treatment of patients with panic disorder. *American Journal of Psychiatry* **155** (May Suppl):1–34.

Amsterdam, E., C. Carter, R. Holloway & T. Schwenk. 1994. Is it normal worry—or pathologic anxiety? *Patient Care:* 26–29.

Battaglia, M. & A. Ogliar. 2005. Anxiety and panic: from human studies to animal research and back. *Neuroscience and Biobehavioral Reviews* **29**(1): 169–179.

Balch, J., & P. Balch. 1990. Prescription for Nutritional Healing. Avery Publishing Group Inc. Garden City Park, New York.

Bouton, M., S. Mineka & D.H. Barlow. 2001. A modern learning theory perspective on the etiology of panic disorder. *Psychological Review* **108**(1): 4–32.

Burns, D. 1980. Feeling Good: The New Mood Therapy. William Morrow and Company, Inc. New York.

Burns, D. 1989. The Feeling Good Handbook. William Morrow and Company, Inc. New York.

Burns, D. 1993. Ten Days to Self-Esteem: The Leader's Manual. William Morrow and Company, Inc. New York.

Childress, A., & D. Burns. 1981. The basics of cognitive therapy. *Psychosomatics* **12**: 1017–1027.

Clark, D. 1986. A cognitive approach to panic. *Behavior Research and Therapy* **4**: 461–470.

Gelder, M. 1983. Is cognitive therapy effective?: Discussion paper. *Journal of the Royal Society of Medicine* **11**: 938–942.

Landon, T.M. & H. Barlow. 2004. Cognitive-behavioral treatment for panic disorder: current status. *Journal of Psychiatric Practice* **10**(4): 211–226.

National Institute of Mental Health. 1993. Panic Disorder in the Medical Setting. By W. Katon. NIH Publication No. 93-3482. Supt. of Docs., U.S. Govt. Printing Office. Washington, DC.

Ninan, P.T. & W. Dunlop. 2005. Neurobiology and etiology of panic disorder. *Journal of Clinical Psychiatry* **66** (Suppl 4): 3–7.

Nutt, D.J. 2005. Overview of diagnosis and drug treatments of anxiety disorders. *CNS Spectrums* **10** (1): 49–56

Otto, M., M. Pollack, S. Meltzer-Brody & J.F. Rosenbaum. 1992. Cognitive-behavioral therapy for benzodiazepine discontinuation in panic disorder patients. *Psychopharmacology Bulletin* **28**(2): 123–130.

Otto, M. & C. Deveney. 2005. Cognitive-behavioral therapy and the treatment of panic disorder: efficacy and strategies. *The Journal of Clinical Psychiatry* **66** (Suppl 4): 28–32.

Rapp, M. 1980. Cognitive therapy: An early appraisal. *Canadian Journal of Psychiatry* **25:** 332–337.

Rayburn, N.R. & W. Otto. 2003. Cognitive-behavioral therapy for panic disorder: A review of treatment elements, strategies, and outcomes. *CNS Spectrums* **8**(5): 356–362.

Roth, W.T. 2005. Physiological markers for anxiety: panic disorder and phobias. *International Journal of Psychophysiology* **58**(2-3): 190–198.

8

Starting a Support Group

"Living with MVPS isn't easy. I wish I had others to talk to who understand. Is there a support group in my area?"

"I want to start a support group. How do I begin? Can you help?"

These are common questions from MVPers. During the past few years many MVPS support groups started—some continue to meet monthly, while others have disbanded. Although support groups are not for everyone, many MVPers enjoy participating. When members of support groups were asked to rank-order their reasons for attending, the number one reason was, "I want more information about MVPS." Other reasons included: "I want to learn how to cope with MVPS symptoms," "I want to talk to others who understand MVPS symptoms," "I believe that only a person with MVPS symptoms can truly understand how I feel," "My symptoms frighten me," "I enjoy helping others help themselves."

What is a Support Group?

A support group is a self-help group that brings together individuals with common goals and concerns. Within the group, members learn they're not alone—that their fears, feelings, and hopes aren't the exception, they're the rule. Meeting together encourages problem-solving by an individual or by a group. When people share, they learn from one another. They gain new insights, become more confident, and enjoy a feeling of accomplishment.

Led by and for their members, these groups are also described as mutual-help groups, and hundreds already exist for a variety of reasons. Keep in mind that it took people with a little bit of courage, a sense of commitment, and a lot of caring to start each group. Examples of such groups include Alcoholics Anonymous, Mended Hearts, and Parents without Partners.

A support group need not meet indefinitely. For example, you may meet a specific goal within a short period of time. On the other hand, a support group may continue for years with different members entering and leaving as their needs change.

Never lose sight, however, of the fact that no support group can meet *all the needs, wants, and desires of all of its members all of the time.* Furthermore, MVP self-help groups are certainly not designed to be psychotherapy groups. Groups with a psychotherapeutic focus require professional leaders with special training.

How Does Someone Start a Support Group?

Who starts an MVP support group? YOU do. If you were not born a support-group leader, you *can* become one. Furthermore, you need not reinvent the wheel. Instead, learn from others who have done it before. Many cities have health-related, self-help support groups. To locate them check with your local self-help clearing-house or the help lines serving your area. Review community papers for time, date, and place of support group meetings. Attend meetings, and speak with the leaders. If you're unable to find a local group, call an MVP support group listed at the end of the chapter.

Benefit from the groups' successes and failures. By doing so, gain confidence, and decide to start a support group. Write for starter packets or any other helpful materials. Be sure to enclose a large, self-addressed and adequately stamped envelope. Many groups work on a tight budget.

Spread the word in your community. How? Contact church groups, civic groups, and school administrators. Post fliers in busy places such as grocery stores, libraries, beauty shops, barber shops, bingo halls. Don't worry about reaching people without MVPS—they may have friends who are looking for a group like yours. Fliers need to simply state, "Looking for energetic people to help start a support group for those with Mitral Valve Prolapse Syndrome. Call (give phone number) between (give time) 5:00 PM and 9:00 PM."

In response to calls, clearly state your expectations. Ask callers if they agree to participate in discussions and share their experiences with MVPS. Will they also involve themselves and help on committees? Some people enthusiastically volunteer to help start a support group and share responsibilities. Others wait for someone else to take over. Don't despair.

Instead, seek help from friends or from health-care professionals sensitive to your needs. For example, contact nurses in cardiologists' offices. If unable to participate, they may refer you to someone else who is knowledgeable and available.

Call the editor of your local newspaper. Ask whether or not he or she publishes announcements of meetings within the community and without charge. If so, say you're interested because you are starting an MVPS support group in the area.

To spark the editor's interest and to possibly get a feature story published, *briefly* explain that MVPS sometimes mimics a full-blown heart attack; it is sometimes misdiagnosed; and it is often a traumatic experience. Invite a reporter to attend a meeting, and offer to lend him this book for additional information.

Provided you do publish notices of meetings, keep them simple. Example: "Please attend a support-group meeting for people with Mitral Valve Prolapse Syndrome, **date, time, specific place and address. Phone (give number)** from 5:00 PM to 9:00 PM **(give appropriate time when someone will be available)**.

Example of a printed flier:

Do you, too, suffer with
Mitral Valve Prolapse Syndrome?
Join others at a first
Support-Group Meeting

DATE: May 8th

TIME: 6:00 P.M.

LOCATION: Mighty Valuable Players' House
                   The Tor Room
                   1968 Taconic Road
                   River Park, NY 12345

For further information call Lisa before 8:00 P.M. at
(321) 232-4753

Carefully read this chapter for suggestions, but use it as only a guide about group dynamics, leadership, problem solving, and more—see references at the end of this chapter.

How Do I Organize and Conduct the First Meeting?

Choose a date and time—preferably evening—that doesn't pose a serious conflict. Review community, school, college, and professional sports calendars. Check newspapers for local events. Even an eager person may find it difficult to attend a meeting during final exams or on baseball's opening day. Later on, should members prefer to change the dates and time of meetings, follow the wishes of the majority.

Select a meeting place in a convenient location—preferably a place that's free of charge. As a suggestion—inquire at a mall, school, church, synagogue, YMCA or YWCA, hospital, university, library, or community center. If you anticipate a small group, have the first meeting in someone's home. Be certain the meeting place is easily accessible and that its location promotes a sense of security or well-being.

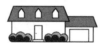

As a group leader, arrive ahead of time. Place chairs in a circle, *without* a special chair for the leader.

Be a good hostess. As people arrive, make them feel welcome. Provide blank stick-on tags and a dry-mark pen for name tags. Direct them to refreshments, and to the meeting area. Also, indicate where rest rooms are located. Keep an attendance book with names, addresses, and telephone numbers. Ask each attendant to regularly sign in.

To begin the meeting, introduce yourself. Then say, "Take a partner—not your spouse or your good friend—but someone you don't already know. Interview each other during the next five minutes and get acquainted." Then ask partners around the circle to introduce *each other*. As each one acknowledges the introduction, ask her to briefly tell something about herself. Allow one or two minutes for each introduction.

What Are the Group Leader's Responsibilities?

The group leader plays an important role. Members with no group experiences look to the leader as a role model—one who sets an example of expected behavior within the group. Members' opinions about a leader are largely based upon her actions. For that reason, a few tips are in order.

1. Be sensitive to others' feelings. The group aims to promote the discovery, expression, and sharing of feelings. The leader encourages others to share their feelings for a reasonable length of time and doesn't interrupt or take control.

2. Avoid a tendency to dominate the group—to think your way is the only way. Remember, this is a support group—not a support person. To encourage each member's participation, emphasize the importance of each one's contribution.

3. Summarize topics that are emphasized, and comment on how the group discussion is going. Your statement should frequently include a question that can facilitate further discussion such as: "Many of you mentioned your frustrations about physicians who dismiss your symptoms as unimportant. Has anyone else had a different experience?

   "Too, I noticed we spent the major portion of the meeting discussing how we manage chest pains and palpitations. Has this been helpful, or would you like to discuss another topic?"

4. Keep members of the group actively involved. Ask a question of anyone who hasn't spoken. Examples: "Peggy, we have not heard from you. How has your week been?

   "Mark, I'm interested in your reaction to what Sarah just described. What has been your experience?"

On the other hand, what do you say to persons who monopolize the conversation and annoy the group? Take a direct and firm approach, for example, "Sue, what you say is important. Now, let us hear from other group members and get *their* opinions." "Bob, your experience is interesting and helpful. Thank you. I sense other members want to add to the discussion, and we encourage each one of you to contribute." (If no one volunteers, ask a question and call upon someone.)

Be prepared for the disruptive or negative member who says something like "What's the use of talking about it? I hear the same complaint over and over."

Remind this person it's what *he* or *she* brings to the group and expresses that generates power. Each member is responsible for his or her own contributions.

Show respect for people's personal commitments. Always begin and end meetings on time. Members may be justifiably angry if they've moved mountains to be punctual and meetings both begin and end late. Furthermore, people may feel compelled to stay later than planned, or feel uncomfortable leaving before everyone else.

Ten or fifteen minutes before closing, let members know the meeting is soon ending. Example: "Since it's almost 8:00 P.M., does anyone have a question, or does anyone wish to quickly discuss something?" This is a good time to recap issues, take care of unfinished business, and announce time and place of the next meeting.

What Are Members Responsibilities?

- Arrive on time.
- Understand the purpose and objectives of the group.
- Listen to and show respect for other people's experiences.
- Encourage others to speak. Don't dominate the group.
- Respect all confidential information.
- Own your feelings. Use the pronoun I—not we—when you talk about yourself.
- Share the responsibility for making the group work

How Do I Keep the Group Going Well for an Extended Period of Time?

First, establish purpose, goals, and objectives.

How often, how long, and when should a support group meet? A support group may meet weekly, semimonthly, or monthly from one to two hours depending upon the group's immediate needs. Keep in mind that enthusiasm is often short-lived, and weekly meetings sometimes quickly lead to burnout.

The support group of the MVP Program of Cincinnati meets the third Wednesday of the month. The first meting in 1988 was an hour long, and—at members' requests—changed to one-and-a-half hours. It works well for us.

To decide *when* to schedule meetings, select a day and a time that is convenient for the majority of members. Propose a week night or a non-traditional time such as a Saturday brunch. A brunch may enable mothers with baby-sitter problems and any-one who doesn't drive at night to attend. Be flexible.

Identify goals of the group. Are goals short-term or long-term?

What are *your* needs and concerns? Within this group which concerns do we commonly share? Why did *you* come to this meeting? (On a flip chart, write members' responses for refer-ence. As a leader, be cautious. Do not assume that *you* know all the needs. Remember, all answers are neither right nor wrong and are worthy of discussion.)

Follow through, therefore, and discuss members' concerns to determine additional objectives. You may always add more as you go along. Write all objectives as *positive statements* such as: Through this group we'll learn how to deal with our fears. Together we aim to better educate the public about MVPS. We shall share as much information as possible from lectures, from journals, and from this book.

Periodically review objectives. Note any changes in focus within the original group and promptly act. What first began as a sharing of information by members may change. Now, mem-bers may wish to become better informed though lectures by knowledgeable people in the medical field. In any event, be alert to the group's wishes. Act accordingly, and don't allow the group to stagnate.

Determine acceptable ground rules.

Be sure that all rules are clear and agreeable to each mem-ber. For example: Everyone has a right to speak while others politely listen without interrupting. Every speaker rightfully expects confidentiality within the group. We succeed only if *we trust each other.* This is extremely important. Let there be no misconceptions regarding the group's purpose.

Encourage input from all members—both new and old

Remember to always welcome new members. Ask them to introduce themselves and briefly tell when they were first diagnosed, what symptoms they have, and how they help themselves. Expect some to say, "Gosh, does that sound familiar."

Be careful, however, to avoid the pitfall of the core-group members becoming a clique. The welcoming of new members is a process that continues well beyond welcoming them at the door. Consider a follow-up phone call to new members. How did they like the meeting? Do they plan on attending again? If not, why?

In time, the support group becomes a combination of new and old members; that's good. New members benefit from long-term members' experiences. Likewise, long-term members benefit by learning about recent practices and procedures from new members.

Invite long-term members who are symptom-free—and who otherwise may drop out—to remain active and serve as role models. By all means, try to involve them as group facilitators. Ask them to speak at meetings and offer suggestions based upon their own experiences. Members attentively listen to someone who has already "walked in *their* shoes."

Encourage discussion. Ask questions to help members share, think about, and learn from each other's experiences and insights.

EXAMPLES

Who were most supportive to me in helping me deal with MVPS? What have they said or done that helps me the most?

Who were least supportive? What have they said or done that has not helped?

What should I say in a note or a letter to someone who is facing what I faced?

What is the worst problem that I must face with MVPS?

What problems related to MVPS have I faced and overcome? What problems have I failed to deal with and why?

How did MVPS control my life? In what ways have I learned how to take control.

If I have learned something special about life or human nature as a result of my situation, what is it?

Ensure a Sense of Belonging—Form Committees

Prepare a list of proposed committees on a flip chart. Leave enough free space underneath each one to write names. Briefly discuss the duties of each committee, length of time each committee serves, and rotation of responsibilities.

Next, either alphabetically assign members to each committee, or ask for volunteers. (To *assign* members may be more effective—we all know the "let-George-do-it" type.) Do remember, however, to ensure the group's success by seeing that each member feels needed and respected. Therefore, encourage each one to assume some responsibility as a committee member. As a group leader, carefully choose a chairperson of each committee—someone who appears to be outgoing and responsible.

Finance committee

You'll need money for postage, paper, refreshments, and other incidentals. Dues may be necessary, but don't assume everyone can afford to pay. It's possible, therefore, that you may solicit donations from a local organization or business. Examples: A supermarket or a bakery may donate snacks. A printing place may donate scrap paper for fliers.

Recruitment and retention committee

To encourage attendance, telephone each member at least one week before every meeting. Ask whether or not each member plans to attend. Then, notify the refreshment committee about how many to prepare for. On the other hand, be prepared to contact members when meetings are canceled. A telephone tree is helpful. Sally calls two members; these two call two others, and so on.

Develop a phone network or an *MVP Hotline*. Encourage the exchange of telephone numbers to provide members with help by phone when it's needed between meetings. Be certain to include the time of day each member can be called.

To recruit new members, continue to spread the word. Post fliers and advertise in local papers. Be careful, however, to prevent burnout or undue stress on any one member. List *two* contact persons on all publicity material. This is particularly true for groups who receive many calls.

Refreshment committee

Solicit food and beverages from members on a rotating basis. Remind members to bring appropriate foods—no caffeinated beverages or chocolate-glazed doughnuts.

Expect the group to experience regular ups and downs in both attendance and enthusiasm. It's natural and to be expected. You'll find this to be true particularly during summer months. Consider meeting every other month, and return to monthly meetings in the fall.

As group leader you may want to join or form a coalition or association of leaders from the same or similar types of self-help groups, for mutual support and for sharing successful program ideas.

How Do I Terminate a Support Group?

Expect the life spans of support groups to vary. Some groups at their inception specify a definite number of weeks or months in which to achieve their objectives. For them, termination is expected and accepted.

On the other hand, some groups form stronger bonds and continue to meet month after month, year after year. For these members, the thought of disbanding sometimes poses problems.

Either way, ending need not be a gloomy affair. Instead, let it signal a new *beginning*. Now that you better understand MVPS, you deal with it, and you take control.

Keep in mind that you want members to leave with a sense of satisfaction and closure. At the last meeting, therefore, review and discuss original objectives. Next, evaluate accomplishments versus shortcomings.

For example, ask yourselves the following questions. What progress have you made as an individual or as a group? What have you learned from each other? How did you feel when you first attended a meeting? How do you feel now? What concerns do you still have? Can you cope with MVPS more satisfactorily? If so, in what way? To answer these questions puts your goals in perspective. Thus, you focus on *achievements*.

During the period of termination, remember several house-keeping items. Pay outstanding bills. Return borrowed supplies or equipment. Notify and thank sponsors, referral agencies, and whoever furnished a meeting room, as well as anyone else who helped. Explain that your group accomplished its objectives and terminates on [date]. In this way, you leave the door open for future groups who may wish to be accommodated.

Finally, when your group disbands, write the names, addresses, and phone numbers of newly made friends. Keep in touch. For, as a song popular during the 1960's goes:

"I get by with a little help from my friends."

See Chapter 11 for MVPS Support Groups

References

Govaerts, K. 1991. Starting a support group. *Diabetes Forecast* 54–60.

Nichols, K. & J. Jenkinson. 1991. Leading a Support Group. Chapman and Hall. London.

Scordo, K. 2001. Factors associated with participation in a mitral valve prolapse support group. *Heart & Lung* **30:** 128–137.

Scordo, K. 2000. The treatment of mitral valve prolapse syndrome in an out-patient nurse-managed MVP clinic. *Nursing Clinics of North America* **35:** 1005–1017.

Scordo, K. 1998. Mitral valve prolapse syndrome: Interventions for symptom control. *Dimensions of Critical Care Nursing* **17:** 177–186.

Scordo, K. 1997. Mitral valve prolapse syndrome: Nonpharmacologic management. *Critical Care Nursing Clinics of North America* **9:** 555–564.

Toseland, R., & R. Rivas. 1984. An Introduction to Group Work Practice. Macmillan. New York.

Utz, S.W. 1994. Helful hints for facilitating suport groups. Personal communication.

White, B. & E. Madara. 1992. The Self-Help Sourcebook: Finding & Forming Mutal Aid Self-Help Groups, 4th ed. St. Clare's-Riverside Medical Center. Denville, NJ.

9

Medication for MVPS

The purpose of this chapter is to *briefly* highlight information about medications commonly used with MVPS. The intent is not to recommend one drug over another, or indeed to recommend any medication. In fact, many MVPers do well *without* medications, while others *require* medication for symptom control. Therefore, *always* discuss the need for medication with your health-care provider.

Remember, medications don't *cure* MVPS. Unlike a kidney infection, for which you take an antibiotic to effect a *cure*, medication for MVPS is prescribed *to lessen the intensity, or frequency of debilitating symptoms*. For example: Some MVPers take medication for frequent palpitations that cause syncope—temporary loss of consciousness. Others take medication to prevent migraine headaches. Many MVPers take prescribed beta-blockers to relieve chest pains and palpitations, others don't.

In spite of beta-blockers, some taking beta-blockers continue to be symptomatic. In the MVPS Health Concerns study, 40% of the participants took one or more medications for MVPS symptoms. The majority of these individuals took a beta blocker and/or anxiolytic agent, while a few others took digoxin or a calcium channel blocker. Analysis of the data suggested that despite medication, the majority of those persons continued to be symptomatic. Many participants in this study were symptom-free and on no medications. That is, despite not using any medications, they were asymptomatic, while others who took medications continued with symptoms. Although reasons for this are likely multifactorial, data thus far suggest that medications given specifically for MVPS may have little effect on symptoms.

A complete list of medications, side effects, and drug interactions, are beyond the scope of this book. If you're interested in further information about medication, see references at the end of this chapter or consult your health-care provider. For a discussion of medications used for the treatment of anxiety and panic attacks, see Chapter 7.

Beta-Blocking Agents

The group of drugs commonly prescribed for symptomatic MVPS are beta-blockers. These drugs may prevent migraine headaches and may alleviate symptoms such as chest pain and palpitations.

As you learned in Chapter 1, catecholamines (epinephrine, norepinephrine) regulate many bodily responses. Effects of catecholamines depend upon their interactions with specific receptors located on cell membranes. Receptors recognize catecholamines, allow these substances to interact with the cell, and cause varying physiological responses.

To simplify an explanation of how catecholamines interact to regulate bodily responses, consider the following analogy.

Your daughter's new date—norepinephrine—comes to your house—a cell. Norepinephrine rings the doorbell. You let him in, since you are a receptor and as a receptor, you recognize a catecholamine. One look at this scruffy character—norepinephrine—and you faint. He caused a physiological response in you, the receptor.

Two types of receptors within the sympathetic nervous system are alpha and beta. Alpha receptors are located in blood vessels throughout the body. Stimulation of alpha receptors by catecholamines (epinephrine and norepinephrine) causes constriction or narrowing of blood vessels. Beta receptors are

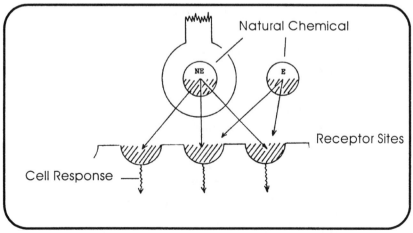

NATURAL CHEMICALS: NE-NOREPINEPHRINE; E-EPINEPHRINE

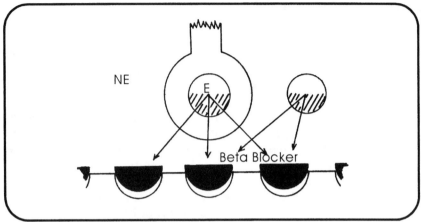

BETA BLOCKER

divided into the beta$_1$-receptors found in heart muscle, and the beta$_2$-receptors found in the heart muscle and the bronchial (lung) and vascular smooth muscle.

Stimulation of beta receptors in the heart causes an increase in heart rate and strengthens the heart muscle's contraction. Stimulation of receptors in vascular smooth muscle causes blood vessels to dilate. Drugs that *block* the action of these receptors are called *beta-blockers.*

Beta-*blockers* block actions of the sympathetic nervous system—the accelerator. To do this, they block the action of epinephrine and norepinephrine. The pharmacological properties determine the precise action of the drug. Predictable effects of beta-blockers include lowered blood pressure; lowered resting

BETA-BLOCKING AGENTS

- Blockadren (timolol)
- Corgard (nadolol)
- Inderal (propranolol)
- Kerlone (betaxolol)
- Lopressor (metoprolol)
- Sectral (acebutolol)
- Tenormin (atenolol)
- Toprol XL (metoprolol extended release)
- Visken (pindolol)
- Zebeta (bisoprolol fumarate)

heart rate, as well as lowered heart rate response during exercise; a blunting of the sympathetic nervous system's response to stress; an increase in left ventricular volume (amount of blood in the heart's pumping chamber), and a decrease in the force of the heart's contraction.

How do beta-blockers affect your heart rate? Suppose you're physically deconditioned. Your pulse rate at rest is 100 beats per minute. After you climb a flight of stairs, your heart rate increases to 150 beats per minute. Your health-care provider prescribes a beta-blocker. Now your resting heart rate slows to 60 beats per minute. Again, climb the same flight of stairs at the same pace. With a beta-blocker your heart rate increases to *only* 90 rather than 150 beats per minute. Thus, beta-blockers attenuate the heart rate's response to exercise.

Possible side effects of beta-blockers include fatigue, nightmares, mental depression, stomach upset, sexual dysfunction, cold extremities, and wheezing or worsening of asthma. If you experience any of these symptoms, notify your health-care provider.

The peak action of the long-acting beta-blockers—Corgard, Kerlone, Tenormin, Toprol XL, Zebeta—occurs two to four hours after taken. This may cause fatigue and sleepiness. To combat these feelings, take a once-a-day beta-blocker in the *evening.*

Beta-blockers may interact with other medications. Aluminum salts found in some antacids, and cholesterol-lowering medications such as Colestid (colestipol) and Questran (cholestyramine) may decrease the absorption of beta-blockers. Therefore, be *sure* to take these medications at *least two hours* after you take a beta-blocker. Similarly, food may alter the availability of the drug absorbed in the stomach. Therefore, establish a pattern, and regularly take the medication either with or without food. This helps to minimize any variation in absorption.

Digitalis

Digitalis—digoxin, digitoxin, Lanoxin, Lanoxicaps—is usually given to MVPers with arrhythmias such as PSVT (paroxysmal supraventricular tachycardia) and atrial fibrillation. Digitalis slows the heart rate; slows electrical conduction to prevent excessive impulses from being conducted to the ventricles; and strengthens the force of the heart's contraction.

Digitalis preparations have a variety of drug interactions. For example: antacids, bran, antibiotics (neomycin, sulfasalazine) and some cholesterol-lowering agents (Questran, Colestid) decrease the absorption of digitalis. Since these interactions decrease the amount available for the body's use, don't take any of the above-mentioned medications *together.* Instead, take each medication *two hours apart.* On the other hand, some antibiotics (erythromycin and tetracycline) *can increase* the amount of digitalis in the body. Also, many drugs interfere with the excretion of digitalis. *Always notify your health-care provider if any additional medications are ever prescribed for you.*

An initial sign that there's too much digitalis in your system is a loss of appetite sometimes followed by nausea and vomiting. Other side effects may include headache, fatigue, drowsiness, and generalized muscle weakness. If any of these symptoms occur, notify your health-care provider.

Calcium Channel Blockers

To varying degrees, calcium channel blockers affect the heart rate, electrical conduction, and the tone of the arterial and venous blood vessels. From this group of drugs, diltiazem and Verapamil are used primarily for the management of arrhythmias and migraine headaches. Verapamil or diltiazem, either by themselves or in combination with digitalis or beta-blockers,

CALCIUM CHANNEL BLOCKING AGENTS

- Cardizem, Dilacor, Tiazac (diltiazem)
- Cardene (nicardipine)
- DynaCirc (isradipine)
- Isoptin, Verelan, Calan (verapamil)
- Nimotop (nimodipine)
- Norvasc (amlodipine)
- Plendil (felodipine)
- Procardia, Adalat (nifedipine)
- Sular (nisoldipine)
- Vascor (bepridil)

can be helpful in the management of atrial fibrillation or paroxysmal supraventricular tachycardia (PSVT).

These drugs are usually well tolerated, but side effects are
possible. They may include constipation, dizziness, lightheadedness, and swelling of ankles or legs.

Antiarrhythmic Drugs

This group of drugs is used to treat MVPers with ventricular
arrhythmias—abnormalities of the heart's rhythm that originate
from the heart's lower chambers. Before these drugs are used,
two critical questions must be answered. One, is the arrhythmia
serious enough to require therapy?, and two, which specific
drug should be used?

The answer to the first question includes MVPers who have
arrhythmias that cause syncope—temporary loss of consciousness. This small group is usually treated with medication. A
larger group of people experience palpitations or skipped beats.
Although usually benign, the arrhythmia disrupts each one's
general well-being and causes undue anxiety. For these
MVPers, antiarrhythmics may be indicated. Treatment depends
on the type and severity of the arrhythmia. Although beta-
blockers and calcium channel blockers are commonly used,
antiarrhythmics such as Betapace (sotalol), Cordarone (amiodarone), Pacerone (amiodarone) Rythmol (propafenone), or
Tikosyn (dofetilide) may be prescribed.

Orthostatic Hypotension: Fludrocortisone (Florinef® Acetate)

When non-pharmacological methods fail, fludrocortisone may
be prescribed for individuals with persistent orthostatic
hypotension. Fludrocortisone is a synthetic mineralocorticoid.
Mineralocorticoids occur naturally in the body and primarily
serve to maintain sodium, chloride, and water balance. The
principal mode of action of this synthetic mineralocorticoid is to
increase blood volume.

To decrease the stomach upset that may occur with fludrocortisone, take the medication with food or milk in the morning.
If you have been taking fludrocortisone for a few weeks, do not

suddenly stop the medication. You may need a gradual reduction in dosage before you cease taking this drug. Carry medical identification that—in case of an emergency—will alert others that you take fludrocortisone. Contact your health-care provider if you develop dizziness, severe or continuing headaches, swelling of feet or lower legs, unusual weight gain, or signs of an infection. This may necessitate discontinuation or a reduction in dosage of the drug. Remember to stay in contact with your health-care provider, who will also monitor your blood levels of various substances, such as blood sugar and potassium. Potassium supplementations may be required, particularly when higher doses of fludrocortisone are used.

Summary

Because many MVPers are young, and medications have side effects, long-term drug therapy is usually avoided. Most health-care providers recommend that MVPers become more knowledgeable and learn to rely more on non-drug interventions to decrease their symptoms.

Questions Commonly Asked about Medications

1. Do I have to take medication for MVPS for the remainder of my life?

This depends on why the medication was originally prescribed. If, for example, you presently take medication because you have experienced episodes of passing out due to arrhythmia, most likely you must continue the medication. If, however, you take medication for other symptoms—chest pain or headache—you may be able to discontinue it. Many MVPers take medication, particularly a beta-blocker, only prior to and during stressful situations that increase their symptoms. Discuss this with your health-care provider.

Many people experience symptoms even with medications. Others cannot tolerate the side effects of the drug. There are those MVPers who prefer not to take any medication. As one of our MVP Program participants said, "Before I joined the program, I experienced fatigue, extra heart beats, and chest pains. Although I took a beta-blocker, my symptoms continued. Now that I want to get pregnant, I avoid taking any form of medication. Instead, with exercise, proper diet, and relaxation techniques, I weaned myself off the beta-blocker. Furthermore, I even feel better now than I did before."

A note of caution: Do not stop taking any medication until you discuss it with your health-care provider. Also be sure you know *why* each medication is prescribed. For example, will it control chest pains, or is it prescribed for other reasons?

2. What should I ask my physician about my medications?

For various reasons, many MVPers hesitate to question their health-care provider about prescribed medications. "He's too busy. He will think my question is stupid. I'm not sure what to ask." To correctly take a prescribed medication—know *what* you'll take and why, *when* to take it, and whether side effects are possible. Take notes, and don't leave the health-care provider's office till you fully understand. If you think of additional questions later on, write them down and either *call* the health-care provider's office, or *wait* until your next visit.

3. Is it true you can't benefit from exercise if you take a beta-blocker?

MVPers who take beta-blockers often believe they can't obtain a *training effect*—or benefit from cardiovascular exercise—because beta-blockers lower resting rate and exercise heart rate—two indicators of a training effect. This, however, is not entirely true.

You'll recall from Chapter 5 that cardiovascular exercise offers many benefits. The extent of the training effect, however, depends upon many factors. These include your initial level of fitness; type and dosage of beta blocker; and frequency, duration, and intensity of exercise. The results of a graded exercise stress test—proof of effectiveness of cardiovascular training—depend upon whether the initial test and follow-up test were both performed while you took a beta-blocker.

If you take a beta-blocker, don't try to achieve a target heart rate. To increase your heart rate to such a level requires high-intensity exercise. This is unnecessary and not recommended. You'll easily tire, exercise less, and enjoy very little benefit from exercise. Instead, use the Borg scale of perceived exertion, and

PRACTICAL GUIDELINES FOR DRUG TREATMENT

- Take your medications at the same times each day.
- If you miss a dose, do not double the next scheduled dose.
- Carry a list of your medications or a medication card in your wallet or purse.
- List both the trade and generic names of the drugs.
- Before having surgery—including dental surgery, or emergency treatment—notify the health-care provider of your medications.
- If you are either pregnant, or plan to become pregnant, or are breast feeding, let your health-care provider know before you take medications. Medications may have an adverse effect on the fetus. They may also pass into the breast milk and cause unwanted effects in the infant.
- When you travel, carry enough medication with you to last a few days in case your luggage is misplaced; or in the event your trip is unexpectedly lengthened.
- Keep drugs in their original containers to maintain the drugs' potency.
- Keep original labels on the drug's container.
- Store medications in a cool, dry place, out of direct sunlight. A medicine cabinet in a warm, humid bathroom, a glove compartment or a car's trunk—particularly during warmer weather—are *poor* storage places.
- *Never* share prescriptive medications with friends. Others may be allergic to the drug, or they *may not* have the same problem, and react differently.
- Never take medications in darkness because bottles and pills look alike. Serious errors are possible.
- Never swallow medications while lying down.
- Regularly clean out your medication cabinet. Over time, moisture, heat and light degrade medications and render them less active. In some cases, decomposed medication becomes a dangerous drug. Therefore, dispose of outdated drugs, old prescription medications with no expiration dates; unidentifiable medicine; cracked, chipped or discolored tablets; and capsules that have softened, cracked, or stuck together. Flush unsafe medications down the toilet. Never throw them in a waste-paper basket or a garbage pail.
- Don't put more than one medication in a bottle.
- Always ask a pharmacist or other health professional how to take medications. To crush or chew a pill may alter its reaction in the body.
- Always read labels for proper administration of the drug and for drug interactions.

exercise only to a perception of *somewhat hard.* That's sufficient. Although it may take longer to achieve a training effect, *it will happen.*

References

About your Medications. 1986. The United States Pharmacopeial Convention, Inc. Rockville, MD.

Blomström-Lundqvist, C. *et al.* 2003. Management of patients with supraventricular arrhythmias. *Journal of the American College of Cardiology* **42:** 1493–1531.

Boudoulas, H. & C. Wooley. 1988. Mitral valve prolapse syndrome: Therapeutic considerations. *In* Mitral Valve Prolapse and the Mitral Valve Prolapse Syndrome H. Boudoulas & C. Wooley, Eds.: 555–563. Futura Publishing Company. Armonk, New York.

Clayman, C., Ed. 1988. The American Medical Association Guide to Prescription and Over-the-Counter Drugs. Random House. New York.

Dajani, A., K. Taubert, W. Wilson, A. Bolger, A. Bayer, P. Ferrieri, *et al.* 1997. Prevention of bacterial endocarditis. Recommendations by the American Heart Association. *JAMA* **277**(22): 1794–1801.

Freeman, R. 2003. Treatment of orthostatic hypotension. *Seminars in Neurology* **23**(4): 435–442.

Frishman, W. 1984. Clinical Pharmacology of the B-Adrenoceptor Blocking Drugs, 2nd ed. Appleton-Century-Crofts. Norwalk, CT.

Griffin, J., P. D'Arcy & C. Speirs. 1988. A Manual of Adverse Drug Interactions. Wright. London.

Hansten, P. & J. Horn. 1989. Drug Interactions, 6th ed. Lea & Febiger. Philadelphia.

Harvard Medical School Health Letter. March 1989. 14, 5.

Katzung, B., Ed. 1989. Basic and Clinical Pharmacology, 4th ed. Appleton & Lange. Norwalk, CT.

McEvoy, G., Ed. 1990. American Hospital Formulary Service Drug Information 90. American Society of Hospital Pharmacists, Inc. Bethesda, MD.

Opie, L., Ed. 1991. Drugs for the Heart, 3rd ed. Grune & Stratton, Inc. New York.

Reiser, J. & L. Horowitz, Eds. 1985. Mechanisms and Treatment of Cardiac Arrhythmias: Relevance of Basic Studies to Clinical Management. Urban & Schwarzenberg. Baltimore-Munich.

Saltissi, S. *et al.* 1983. The effects of oral digoxin therapy in primary mitral leaflet prolapse. *European Heart Journal* **4:** 828–837.

Scordo, K. 2007. Medication use and symptoms in individuals with mitral valve prolapse syndrome. *Clinical Nursing Research* **16**(1). In press.

10

Herbal Therapy and MVPS

Many MVPers use complementary or alternative therapy in the form of natural products, including herbal medicine, functional foods (garlic), animal-based (glucosamine) supplements, or dietary supplements (vitamins) to help control symptoms. Many do so because these health-care alternatives are more congruent with their own beliefs, values, and philosophy of health and life. Also, they have found conventional medicine has not been very helpful in symptom control. In the MVP Health Concerns study, commonly used natural products for symptom control included Bach flower remedies, black cohosh, blue-green algae, chamomile, coenzyme Q10, evening primrose oil, garlic, ginkgo biloba, kava, flaxseed, ginseng, hawthorn, omega 3 fatty acid, magnesium (discussed in Chapter 4), St. John's wort, and valerian. Vitamins were mainly multivitamins and vitamin E. The popularity of these products is similar to that found in a recent survey completed by the National Center for Alternative and Complementary Medicine (NCCAM), National Institutes of Health (NIH). According to this survey, the most commonly used natural products were echinacea, ginseng, ginkgo biloba and garlic supplements. Before discussing these therapies, a word of caution is advised.

Although the use of herbal remedies may help control a variety of symptoms, the United States Food and Drug Administrations does not monitor the safety of herbal medication. The Dietary Supplement and Health Education Act of 1994 (DSHEA) assigned the responsibility for ensuring efficacy and safety to the manufacturers of the medication. Studies on safety, side effects and potential drug interactions are costly and, for many manufacturers, cost-prohibitive. There are currently no requirements to submit documentation of testing a product. Thus, limited data are available. Manufacturers, however, must make sure that product label information is truthful and not misleading. They are not allowed to make claims of a cure for a disease, but they may state the physiological effects of the product. For example, a manufacturer can claim that an herbal medication "boosts the immune system" or "strengthens the heart." What are unknown to the consumer are the true contents of the product's active ingredients, fillers, and preservatives, and the effectiveness, safety, adverse reactions, or interactions with other medications. Because dietary supplements are not always tested for manufacturing consistency, even the composition may vary considerably from lot to lot.

In contrast to the United States, herbal medicines have a special status in Germany. The legal basis for modern drug laws in Germany is based on the European Community Directives, initially issued in 1965. Under the terms of these directives all member states of the European Community pledged to establish a formal review of all medicinal products on the market and to assure that they met appropriate standards for quality and purity. Products were to be reviewed for safety and efficacy and re-registered by 1990 in Germany. Consequently, in 1976, Germany passed the Second Medicines Act (Arzneimittelgesetz 1976, or AMG 76), which went into effect January 1, 1978. This act required that the entire range of medicines in the pharmaceutical market—including conventional drugs, as well as medicinal plants and phytomedicines—be reviewed by scientific committees. In 1978 the Minister of Health established a series of commissions (Commission E) comprising physicians, pharmacologists, toxicologists, representatives of the pharmaceutical industry, and lay persons. Commission E evaluated data obtained from clinical trials, research studies, field studies, collections of single cases, and expertise of medical associations. The results were published in the form of monographs in the *Bundesanzeiger*—the German equivalent to the *Federal Register* in the US. *Herbal Medicine: Expanded Commission E Monographs* (2000) is the latest reference that updates the original English translation of the Commission E monographs published by the American Botanical Society in 1998. This book is an excellent resource for individuals who want detailed information on commonly used herbs.

It is important to know that even if an herbal supplement is labeled "natural," it does not mean it is safe or without any harmful effects. For example, the herbs kava and comfrey have been linked to serious liver damage. Ephedra, or ma huang, has been linked to heart attacks, stroke, and cardiovascular collapse. Herbal supplements can act in the same way as drugs. Therefore, they can cause medical problems if used incorrectly or if taken in large amounts. Women who are pregnant or nursing should be especially cautious about using herbal supplements, since these products can act like drugs.

In an attempt to overcome some of these issues, in 1998 the National Center for Complementary and Alternative Medicine (NCCAM) was established by Congress as an office within the National Institutes of Health. Because of budget constraints, only a few of the many herbal medications available have been studied. Although critiquing research studies is beyond the scope of this book, a word to the wise is in order. Two research methods or processes are used to study alternative therapy—*observational* or *interventional.* Interventional research includes planning, developing, implementing, and testing the intervention. Observational research is collecting data by recording and observing activities or behaviors that are related to a particular area of interest. The conclusions of an observational study and those of an interventional study can show two very different outcomes. A good example may be seen in the studies of vitamin E supplements. Observational studies suggested that the use of daily vitamin E daily decreased the risk for the development of cardiovascular disease. Interventional trials, however, reported by the American College of Cardiology and the American Heart Association, concluded that there is no evidence to support the previous findings from observational trials. In essence, association does not prove causation. Conclusions regarding alternative therapies are best drawn from randomized, controlled interventional trials.

This chapter is designed to give the reader a *brief, basic* overview of what is currently known about the herbal products most commonly used by MVPers. *There are currently no controlled research trials that address the use of a specific herbal product in the control of MVPS symptoms, and thus recommendations cannot be made.* For MVPers who wish further information, please see the references at the end of the chapter. Additionally, there are numerous books written about natural products. Remember to consult your health-care provider before using an herbal supplement, especially if you are taking any medications—whether prescription or over-the-counter. Some herbal supplements are known to interact with medications in ways that cause health problems and may worsen, instead of lessen, MVPS symptoms.

Bach Flower Remedies

Bach flower remedies were developed by the English physician Edward Bach during the 1930s on the basis of his belief that mental attitude plays a vital role in maintaining health and recovering from illness. He believed that the remedies contained small amounts of the plant's life-force energy which enabled them to provide vibrational patterns needed to either neutralize or serve as an antidote to negative emotional, behavioral, or cognitive states. A Bach flower remedy consists of water that has been patterned with the energetic vibrations of one of 38 different flowers. The remedy is added to a cup of water (or other beverage) and taken four times a day. Although further research is needed to evaluate this healing modality, the 38 flower tinctures are believed to heal emotional imbalances such as despondency, despair, and fear. MVPers commonly take Bach flower treatment to help control fear, anxiety and insomnia. There is no standard remedy for any one disorder; each person requires a unique treatment. Depending on symptoms, remedies can be used singly or in combinations to a maximum of seven. Flower remedies are not reported to have side effects and do not interfere with other alternative or conventional medicines.

Black Cohosh

(*Actaea racemosa* and *Cimicifuga racemosa*)

Black cohosh is a member of the buttercup family; it is a perennial that is grown in the eastern regions of the United States and parts of Canada. Although this herb has multiple reported uses—as a diuretic, an antispasmodic, an antitussive, an astringent, an antiarthritic, an antidiarrheal and a smooth muscle relaxant—it is primarily used for hot flashes and other menopausal symptoms. Black cohosh influences the endocrine regulatory systems, with effects similar to one of the milder endogenous estrogens, estriol. Many MVPers take this to help control symptoms of PMS (premenstrual syndrome). Because of its low incidence of side effects, in the 2004 position statement on the treatment of menopausal symptoms, the North American Menopause Society (NAMS) recommends the use of black cohosh for no longer than six months—the effects of long-term use are unknown. These authors caution that black cohosh should not be used in women with breast cancer, because the currently available evidence is contradictory.

The recommended dose of black cohosh is 20 mg of Remifemin twice a day for no more than six months. Therapeutic benefits may take from four to twelve weeks. Currently, Remiferemin (SBG-R) is the only commercially prepared black cohosh that has been clinically tested for safety and efficacy. Side effects include hypotension, nausea, vomiting, anorexia, and uterine stimulation. Presently, there are no known herb-to-food or herb-to-herb interactions. Because of a potential risk of low blood pressure, cautiously use black cohosh if you take medications that lower blood pressure. Also, because black cohosh may alter other hormone therapy, be certain to let your health-care provider know if you take this herb along with hormonal therapy. Women with breast cancer may want to avoid black cohosh until its effects on breast tissue are understood.

Blue-Green Algae
(*Spirulina* sp., *Aphanizomenon flos-aquae*)

Blue-green algae grows in lakes, particularly those rich in salts, in Central and South America, and Africa. *Spirulina* species are cultured in alkaline freshwater while *Aphanizomenon flos-aquae* (AFA) is naturally grown and harvested from Upper Klamath Lake, Oregon (USA). Blue-green algae products frequently contain one or both of these strains of algae. Spirulina is a rich source of nutrients, containing up to 70% protein, B-complex vitamins, phycocyanin, chlorophyll, beta-carotene, vitamin E, and numerous minerals. In fact, spirulina contains more beta-carotene than carrots. Spirulina has been used since ancient times as a source of nutrients and has been said to possess a variety of medical uses as an antioxidant, antiviral, antineoplastic, weight loss aid, and lipid-lowering agent. MVPers reportedly take this to help control stress and depression.

Doses used in research studies are as follows: Diabetes mellitus (type 2): 1 gram of spirulina by mouth twice daily with meals; high cholesterol: 1.4 grams of spirulina by mouth, three times daily with meals; oral leukoplakia (pre-cancerous mouth lesions): 1 gram of *Spirulina fusiformis* by mouth daily; and weight loss: 200 milligrams of spirulina tablets by mouth three times daily, taken just before eating.

Frequently reported adverse effects include headache, anorexia, nausea, vomiting, muscle pain, sweating, flushing of the face, and difficulty concentrating. Skin reactions have also been reported. Blue-green algae, especially types that are usually harvested in uncontrolled settings (*Anabaena* spp., *Aphanizomenon* sp., and *Microcystis* sp.), may be contaminated with heavy metals. Liver damage has also been reported. The amino acid phenylalanine in blue-green algae may cause an adverse reaction in people with the genetic condition phenylketonuria (PKU), and should be used cautiously.

Chamomile
(*Matricaria recutita; Chamaemelum nobile*)

Chamomile is a low-growing annual herbaceous plant that is natively found from southern and eastern Europe to northern and western Asia. Chamomile is used to treat inflammation, anxiety, insomnia, and spasms. It has also been used for treatment of digestive disorders such as Crohn's disease, irritable bowel syndrome, indigestion, colitis, and as a topical cream or ointment for wound healing. In the United States, chamomile is best known as an ingredient in herbal tea preparations advertised for mild sedating effects. MVPers take chamomile to help control stress and to facilitate sleep.

German chamomile (*Matricaria recutita*) and Roman chamomile (*Chamaemelum nobile*) are the two major types of chamomile used for health conditions. They are believed to have similar effects on the body, although German chamomile may be slightly stronger. While chamomile is widely used, there is not enough reliable research in humans to support its use for any condition.

Adverse reactions are rare and include allergic reaction and vomiting. Vomiting was reported after large quantities of the dried flowers were ingested. On account of possible hypersensitivity reactions, individuals who are allergic to ragweed, pollen, chrysanthemums, or asters should cautiously use chamomile.

Chamomile (*Chamaemelum*) should not be used during pregnancy or lactation because it is a known abortifacient (causes abortion). No herb-to-food or herb-to-herb reactions are known. Theoretically, chamomile may increase the effects of alcohol, so they should not be taken together. Also there is possible interference of anticoagulants (blood thinners) and chamomile, and of chamomile's increasing the effects of a sedative. Both should be not be used together. There is no recommended dosage for chamomile products. Traditional doses are 3 grams in 150 ml of water three to four times a day.

Coenzyme Q10 (CoQ10 or Ubiquinone)

CoQ10 is a naturally occurring, fat-soluble antioxidant that is found in the mitochondria (energy component of the cell) of the tissues of many organs such as the heart, liver, and kidney. Antioxidants act to protect the body's cells against the effects of free radicals—potentially damaging by-products of energy metabolism. Free radicals damage cells and may contribute to the development of diseases such as cancer and heart disease. CoQ10 is naturally present in a variety of foods. Organ meats such as heart, liver, and kidney as well as in beef, soybean oil, sardines, mackerel and peanuts are particularly high in CoQ10. Coenzyme Q10 acts as a cellular membrane stabilizer and also functions as a cellular antioxidant to protect against free radical damage.

CoQ10 has reported uses in a variety of diseases such as congestive heart failure, angina pectoris, hypertension, heart arrhythmias, diabetes mellitus, Parkinson's disease, and ischemic heart disease. It is commonly used to prevent or alleviate muscle aches that may be associated with cholesterol-lowering medications such as statins (HMG co-reductase inhibitors). MVPers reported that they take CoQ10 to help control palpitations and chest pain, and for a general feeling of well-being.

Adverse side effects include mostly gastrointestinal reactions such as nausea, diarrhea, vomiting, anorexia, and epigastric pain. Other rare side effects include rash, thrombocytopenia (low blood platelets), irritability, dizziness, and headache. At present, no herb-to-food or herb interactions are known. However, CoQ10 may decrease the action of anticoagulants and concurrent use is discouraged.

Dosage for CoQ10 with a minimum of 30 mg daily appears to increase an individual's blood levels of CoQ10. Typical dosage is 100–150 mg every day divided in two to three doses taken with a small amount of food.

Echinacea
(Purple coneflower; Coneflower; American coneflower)

According to the NCCAM survey, echinacea is the most common natural product used in the United States. Echinacea (*Echinacea angustifolia, Echinacea pallida, Echinacea purpurea)* is frequently used alone or in combination with other herbs to treat or prevent colds, flu, and other upper respiratory infections. Less commonly, echinacea is used to heal wound and skin problems such as acne or boils. Although it is commonly thought of as an immune system stimulant, echinacea might actually have anti-inflammatory effects. Some studies show that echinacea can reduce symptom severity and duration by 10% to 30% if taken within the first few hours after symptoms appear, whereas other studies indicate that echinacea is similar to placebo in preventing colds and other infections.

Echinacea appears to be safe for short-term use. It can cause gastrointestinal side affects and, occasionally, rash. Echinacea is in the same botanical family as ragweed. Thus, individuals with allergic conditions such as asthma, eczema, and allergic rhinitis should avoid echinacea. Because of possible immuno-suppressant effects of echinacea, individuals with autoimmune disorders such as rheumatoid arthritis, multiple sclerosis, and lupus should avoid echinacea products. Also, individuals who take drugs designed to suppress immunity, such as those taken after organ transplant, should avoid echinacea.

Echinacea products vary widely, making it difficult to determine optimal dosing.

Also, labels can be misleading and not reflect the true amounts of echinacea contained within the product. Some resources recommend using echinacea alone. There is no reliable evidence that remedies that contain goldenseal or other herbs work better than echinacea alone. Frequent handwashing and avoiding people with colds remain the most effective and least expensive alternative to herbal remedies.

Evening Primrose Oil
(*Oenothera biennis* L.; *Primula elatior*)

The evening primrose is a member of the willow herb and fuscsia family and is named for a flower that opens and releases scent in the evening. The seeds of the flower contain oils that are used for therapeutic purposes. Evening primrose oil (EPO) contains an omega-6 essential fatty acid, gamma-linolenic acid (GLA), believed to be the active ingredient. Although EPO has been studied in a wide variety of disorders, quality research is lacking. Evening primrose oil has been used to decrease the risk of heart disease by lowering cholesterol and to decrease the risk of blood clots (decreased platelet aggregation). It has also been used for controlling symptoms of premenstrual syndrome (PMS), to reduce breast pain, to decrease symptoms of cystic breast disease as well as for skin conditions (eczema). MVPers take evening primrose oil to help control anxiety and PMS symptoms.

Dosages used in research studies for the treatment of eczema or atopic dermatitis were 4 to 8 grams of evening primrose oil (EPO) daily, taken by mouth, in divided dosages, and for the treatment of breast pain, 3 grams EPO daily, taken by mouth, in divided doses.

On account of the potential of EPO to lower the seizure threshold in individuals with a seizure disorder, avoid EPO if you have a diagnosis of seizures. Adverse reactions include headaches, anorexia, nausea, vomiting, diarrhea, rash, and, with long-term use, immunosuppression.

Flaxseed (*Linum usitatissimum*)

Flaxseed is a blue flowering crop that produces small, flat golden yellow to reddish brown seeds. It is found in United States, Europe, and Canada. Flaxseed and its derivatives (flaxseed oil/linseed oil) are rich sources of the essential fatty acid alpha-linolenic acid, which is a biologic precursor to omega-3 fatty acids. Although omega-3 fatty acids have been associated with improved cardiovascular outcomes, evidence from human trials is mixed regarding the efficacy of flaxseed products for coronary artery disease or hyperlipidemia. As a source of fiber, oral flaxseed (not flaxseed oil) possesses laxative properties, a reason why MVPers take flaxseed. They also find flaxseed to help with irritable bowel symptoms.

Flaxseed oil contains only the alpha-linolenic acid component of flaxseed, and not the fiber or lignan components. Therefore, flaxseed oil may share the purported lipid-lowering properties of flaxseed, but not the proposed laxative or anti-cancer abilities.

Interactions of flaxseed with other medications include decreased absorption. Also flaxseed may increase the action of laxatives and cause diarrhea. Side effects include anorexia, nausea, vomiting, diarrhea, and flatulence. In large doses, or when taken with inadequate water, flaxseed may precipitate bowel obstruction via a mass effect. The effects of flaxseed on blood glucose levels are not clear, although hyperglycemic effects have been reported in one case series. Preliminary evidence suggests that alpha-linolenic acid may be associated with an increased risk of prostate cancer.

Flaxseed can be added to baked products as a whole seed, but it must be ground (milled) prior to consumption to obtain the potential health benefits from the omega-3 fatty acids and lignans. Grind flaxseed using an inexpensive coffee grinder or blender. Store flaxseed in a cool, dry location away from bright light. The recommended dose for constipation is 1 tablespoon of whole or "bruised" seed (not ground) with 150 ml of liquid 2–3 times daily, or 2–3 tablespoons of ground flaxseed for the preparation of flaxseed mucilage (gums). Flaxseed is high in mucilage and if not take with sufficient liquid may lead to a bowel obstruction from a mass effect. Therefore, always take 10 times the amount of water for the amount of flaxseed taken. For lowering cholesterol, the dose is one to two ounces that can be incorporated into breads or muffins. (One ounce (28.4 g) of flaxseed contains more than 5 grams of alpha linoleic acid.)

Unless otherwise instructed by your health-care provider, avoid flaxseed if you have diarrhea, an ileus, a bowel obstruction or narrowing of the esophagus or intestine. Due to possible estrogen-like effects of flaxseed (not flaxseed oil), cautiously use flaxseed if you have a hormone-sensitive condition such as endometriosis, polycystic ovary syndrome, uterine fibroids, or cancer of the breast, uterus, or ovary. Also, caution is advised in individuals with bleeding disorders, those that take blood-thinning medications, and those who plan to undergo medical, surgical, or dental procedures. As with any other mucilage, the absorption of other drugs may be negatively affected.

Garlic (*Allium sativum*)

Garlic—one of the oldest herbal remedies—is the edible bulb from a plant in the lily family. Garlic, onions, leeks, scallions, shallots, and chives are classified as members of the *Allium* genus. Thus, they are commonly described as *Allium* vegetables. Garlic is used as an antiasthmatic, anti-inflammatory and anti-microbial. Although there is conflicting evidence, garlic has the potential to reduce the risk of developing atherosclerosis by reducing blood pressure, lowering lipid and cholesterol levels, and by reducing the stickiness of blood platelets. Also, garlic is claimed to improve glycemic (blood sugar) control, either by increasing the release of insulin or enhancing the response to insulin.

The effects of garlic are primarily attributed to the sulfur-containing compounds, particularly allicin and its transformation products. When raw garlic is cut or crushed, the enzyme allinase interacts with the cysteine compound alliin to produce allicin. This gives the garlic aroma and medicinal properties.

Garlic may cause stomach upset or irritation in some individuals during the initiation of therapy. Additional side effects include bloating, headache, sweating, lightheadedness, menorrhagia (heavy menstrual bleeding) and, of course, garlic odor. Garlic may decrease the effectiveness of certain drugs used to treat HIV (human immunodeficiency virus) and, therefore, should be avoided by persons taking those drugs. Because of the potential risk of increased bleeding, discontinue garlic one week before surgery. The dose is 0.6 to 1.2 grams of dried powder or 2 to 4 grams for fresh garlic daily (about 1 clove) or enteric-coated tablets, 400 mg 2–3 times/day, equivalent to 1200 mg of fresh garlic.

Ginkgo biloba

Ginkgo biloba is a very hardy tree that is resistant to insects and microorganisms. It is native to Japan and China and is now found in the United States and Europe. It has been used to help individuals with Alzheimer's disease decrease the disturbances of cerebral functioning and peripheral vascular insufficiency.

The dried leaves are used to make ginkgo biloba extract EGb 761. The flavanoid components act as an antioxidant to increase the threshold of blood loss from capillaries and reduce capillary fragility. Although there have been some promising results for memory enhancement, a trial sponsored by the National Institute on Aging of more than 200 healthy adults over age 60 found that ginkgo biloba taken for six weeks did not improve memory. Ginkgo biloba has been shown to improve walking distance in people with peripheral vascular disease.

Side effects with ginkgo biloba are mainly mild gastrointestinal side effects and headaches. Ginkgo toxin (a neurotoxin) may decrease the effectiveness of anticonvulsants and therefore should not be used by individuals with epilepsy. Also, on acount of ginkgo biloba's ability to inhibit platelet-activating factor and because of reports of serious bleeding in people who take aspirin or warfarin (Coumadin), persons on blood-thinners or platelet-inhibitors should avoid ginkgo biloba. Dosage for ginkgo biloba is 40–80 mg up to three times a day.

Kava (*Piper methysticum*)

Kava is from the *Piper methysticum* pepper plant rhizome, which is found in the South Sea islands. Supplements containing the herbal ingredient kava are promoted for relaxation (e.g., to relieve stress, anxiety, and tension), sleeplessness, and menopausal symptoms, and other uses. Kava is also reportedly used as a muscle relaxant and to promote wound healing. It is, however, not without a serious potential side effect.

In March 2002, the Food and Drug Administration (FDA) alerted consumers to the potential of severe liver injury that had been associated with the use of kava-containing dietary supplements. Liver disorders reported in ~25 cases included hepatitis, cirrhosis, and liver failure. Four patients required liver transplants. Although the risk of liver damage appears to be rare, the United States FDA recommends that anyone with a liver disease or liver problems consult their health-care provider before taking kava-containing supplements. MVPers take kava to help control anxiety, although many stated that they discontinued this product for fear of liver damage.

Side effects are mainly seen when kava is taken at high doses for a long period of time. These side effects include increased reflexes of the central nervous system, daytime drowsiness, blurred vision, red eyes, nausea, vomiting, hematuria (blood in the urine), decrease in platelets (cells that help clot blood) and lymphocytes (white blood cells that fight infection), shortness of breath, and hypersensitivity reactions to skin, with skin turning yellow and scaling. Kava may increase the sedative effect of anesthetics, and thus be discontinued at least 24 hours before surgery. Herb-to-herb interactions are unknown. Food increases the absorption of kava. People with major depression or Parkinson's disease should not take kava. Kava, when taken with antiparkinsonian drugs, may increase the symptoms of Parkinson's disease. Kava, when combined with benzodiazepines (including alprazolam), increased the risk for sedation and coma. Also, central nervous system depressants, such as alcohol, benzodiazepines, and barbiturates, in combination with kava may also have additive sedative effects. The doses of standard extract for treatment of anxiety and depression are 45–70 mg of kava lactones three times a day. The doses for sedation are 190–200 mg of kava lactones 60 minutes before bedtime. Even if kava is taken within the recommended doses, there may be an adverse affect on motor reflexes affecting driving judgment and/or operating heavy machinery.

Ginseng (*Panax Ginseng*)

The root of Asian ginseng contains active chemical components called ginsenosides (or panaxosides) that are thought to be responsible for the herb's medicinal properties. The root is dried and used to make tablets or capsules, extracts, and teas, as well as creams or other preparations for external use. Although further research is warranted, Asian ginseng has been found to lower blood glucose and have positive beneficial effects on immune function. Ginseng is used to improve overall well-being, help lessen fatigue, increase physical endurance, and improve ability to cope with stress—all reasons why many MVPers take ginseng.

When taken by mouth, ginseng is usually well tolerated. Some sources suggest that its use be limited to three months because of concerns about the development of side effects. The most common side effects are headaches and sleep and gastrointestinal problems. Ginseng may cause allergic reactions. There have been reports of breast tenderness, menstrual irregularities, and high blood pressure associated with ginseng products. The problem, however, is that these products' components were not analyzed, and thus effects may have been due to another herb or drug in the product. Side effects of ginseng may include hypertension, palpitations, chest pain, and in high doses insomnia, anxiety, restlessness, nausea, diarrhea, and vomiting. On account of additive effect of overstimulation, avoid taking ginseng with caffeinated coffee, tea, or cola. One herb-to-herb interaction was noted when ginseng is taken with ephedra; there is an increase in central nervous system stimulation and an increase in hypertension. Ginseng may decrease the action of anticoagulants such as heparin and warfarin. If ginseng is taken concurrently with MAOIs (monoamine oxidase inhibitors), the individual may experience a manic-like syndrome. Because of the known results of ginseng's reducing blood glucose levels, caution is advised if you take oral antidiabetics or insulin since there is a possibility of hypoglycemia.

There are over 54 ginseng products available and 85% of them contain little or no ginseng. Even some American versions contain a high percentage of alcohol, and may contain geranium. Daily average dose is 1 to 2 grams of root in an infusion up to three to four times a day for three to four weeks. For cognitive function, the dose is 400 mg daily. The dosage for effectiveness of hypoglycemic effects in individuals with diabetes is 100–200 mg. To increase oxygen capacity, improve stamina, and reduce stress, 100 mg twice a day is recommended. Because of its hypoglycemic effects and the potential increased risk of bleeding, ginseng should be discontinued at least seven days before surgery.

Hawthorn

Hawthorn (*Crataegus* species), a member of the rose family, was hung over the doorway in the Middle Ages to prevent the entry of evil spirits. The plant is a common thorny shrub that grows up to 5 feet tall on hillsides and in sunny wooded areas throughout the world. Hawthorn rates high as one of the most commonly used herbs. Considered a "cardiotonic" herb, the flowers and berries of the hawthorn plant have been used in traditional medicine to treat irregular heartbeat, high blood pressure, chest pain, hardening of the arteries, and congestive heart failure, with some research to support its benefits. MVPers commonly take hawthorn to help control chest discomfort.

Adverse reactions includes arrhythmias, anorexia (loss of appetite), fatigue, hypotension, nausea, vomiting, sedation, and skin hypersensitivity reactions. There are no known herb-to-food interactions. Interactions with herb-to-other herbals include increased effects of both *Adonis vernalis* (Adonis) and *Convallaria majalis* (lily of the valley), when taken with hawthorn. Herbal to drug interactions include increased risk of hypotension (low blood pressure) when hawthorn is taken with antihypertensives such as beta-blockers. Other interactions include possible increased effort of cardiac glycosides (Lanoxin, digoxin) when taken with hawthorn, and increased sedative effect of the central nervous system when taken with barbiturates, alcohol, and psychotropics. Adult dosage is 160 to 900 mg standardized (4 to 20 mg flavonoids/30 to 160 mg oligomeric procyanidins) fluid crude extract daily for at least six weeks; or 120 to 240 mg extract standardized to 1.8% vitexin rhamnoside/10% procyanidins three times per day for at least six weeks.

Omega-3 Fatty Acid

Interest in fish oil comes from observations 30 years ago of Greenland Eskimos who, despite a very high fat diet, had very low rates of heart disease. This observation sparked numerous studies and is considered by some to be one of the most important advances in the nutritional treatment of heart disease.

Omega-3 fatty acids, found mainly in fish oils, are believed to be beneficial in a multitude of diseases. Much of the evidence is circumstantial and questionable. There is, however, solid and compelling evidence that two long-chain omega-3 fatty acids—eicosapentaenoic (EPA) and docosahexaenoic acid (DHA)—help prevent coronary heart disease and decrease the incidence of sudden death (presumably from a second heart attack). EPA and DAH possess anti-inflammatory, antiarrhythmic, and anti-thrombotic (increased "stickiness" of blood) properties and are found almost exclusively in seafood. Fish do not produce EPA and DHA. Rather, these oils are synthesized by single-celled marine organisms that fish eat. In general, the oiler the fish, the more EPA and DHA. Fish with high concentrations include: tuna, sardines, salmon, mackerel, and herring.

Omega-3 is also important to reduce the negative impact of another essential type of fatty acid known as omega-6. Omega-6 is found in foods such as eggs, poultry, cereals, vegetable oils, baked goods, and margarine. If omega-6s aren't balanced with sufficient amounts of omega-3s, problems can ensue. Research indicates that high omega-6 fatty acids shift the physiologic state to pro-inflammatory and pro-thrombotic. A third kind of fatty acid, alpha-linolenic acid, is less potent. It comes from soybeans, canola, walnut and flaxseed, and oils made from those beans, nuts, and seeds.

Omega-3 and omega-6 fatty acids are essential for good health, but must be obtained through diet or supplementation—they are not synthesized by the body. Unfortunately, in the United States, there has been an enormous increase in the consumption of omega-6 fatty acids with the increased use of vegetable oils from corn, sunflower seeds, safflower seeds, cottonseed, and soybeans in cooking and processing. To balance this effect requires increased intake of omega-3s. Although the optimum ratio of omega-6 to omega 3 is 3:1, in Western diets this is currently typically 10:1 or 12:1.

The American Heart Association (AHA) recommends 1 gram of EPA/DHA daily for individuals with known heart disease. For individuals without heart disease, the AHA recommends eating a variant of (preferably fatty) fish at least twice a week, or about 500 mgm of EPA/DHA per day. Include oils and foods rich in alpha-linolenic acid (flaxseed, canola and soybean oils; flaxseed and walnuts). Higher levels of EPA/DHA are required for individuals with elevated levels of blood triglycerides and this should be done with the supervision of your health-care provider.

Significant amounts of mercury and other environmental contaminants are concentrated in certain species of fish, such as shark, swordfish, king mackerel, and tilefish. Therefore, the FDA and the EPA (Environmental Protection Agency) advise women who may become pregnant, women who ar pregnant, breastfeeding mothers, and young children to avoid eating some

TABLE 10-1. MERCURY AND OMEGA-3 FATTY ACID CONTENT OF FISH

	MEAN MERCURY LEVEL IN PARTS PER MILLION (PPM)	OMEGA-3 FATTY ACIDS (GRAMS PER 3-OZ. SERVING)
FISH WITH THE LOWER LEVELS OF MERCURY		
Canned tuna (light)	0.12	0.26–0.73
Shrimp	ND*	0.27
Pollock	0.06	0.46
Salmon (fresh, frozen)	0.01	0.68–1.83
Cod	0.11	0.13–0.24
Catfish	0.05	0.15–0.20
Clams	ND*	0.24
Flounder or sole	0.05	0.43
Crabs	0.06	0.34–0.40
Scallops	0.05	0.17
Lobster	0.31	0.07–0.41
Grouper	0.55	0.21
Halibut	0.26	0.40–1.00
Oysters	ND*	0.37–1.17
Mahi-mahi	0.19	0.12
Herring	0.04	1.71–1.81
FISH WITH ABOUT 0.5 PPM HG		
Fresh or frozen tuna	0.38	0.24–1.28
Red snapper	0.60	0.27
Orange roughy	0.54	0.002
FISH WITH THE HIGHEST LEVELS OF MERCURY (ABOUT 1 PPM HG)		
Shark	0.99	0.90
Swordfish	0.97	0.70
Tilefish (golden bass or golden snapper)	1.45	0.80
King mackerel	0.73	0.34

*ND, mercury concentration below the level of detection (LOD = 0.01ppm)
Available at: http://www.americanheart.org/presenter.jhtml?identifier=3013797
Accessed January 29, 2006.

types of fish and to eat fish and shellfish that are lower in mercury.

Fish oil capsules vary widely in amounts and ratios of EPA and DHA. A recent *Consumer Reports* noted that to obtain approximately one gram total of EPA/DHA, depending upon the manufacturer, two to five pills are required. The first, and currently only U.S. Food and Drug Administration (FDA)–approved fish oil prescription omega-3 product is Omacor® (Reliant Pharmaceuticals). Each 1-gram capsule contains 90% omega-3-fatty acid (EPA 460 mg and DHA 380 mg.) Omacor is approved by the FDA as an adjunct to diet for people with high triglycerides. Individuals who have a known sensitivity or allergy to shell fish should exercise caution when using fish oil capsules. Omacor® does not contain shell fish; it is made from mackerel, anchovies and sardines. Although there have been no reports of bleeding with Omacor, if you take an anticoagulant such as warfarin (Coumadin®) you should report any signs of excessive bleeding.

Many individuals worry that fish oil capsules contain mercury. This is not true. Mercury is water-soluble, not oil-soluble. When the oil is extracted from the fish, the mercury and other heavy metals stay behind in the fish meal.

Both wild and farmed fish are good sources of omega-3. If farm-fed fish are fed proper diets of fish protein, fish oil, or algae, they will have a high content of omega-3 fatty acids. If they are fed wheat and corn, they won't contain as much. The omega-3 content of wild fish may be more unpredictable—it depends on the maturity of the fish and when it was caught. Also, some researchers report higher amounts of organic pollutants in farmed fish (salmon).

Don't confuse omega-3s with cod liver oil. Cod liver oil comes from the liver, whereas fish oil comes from the body of the fish. Cod liver oil is very high in vitamin A. If you take it, be very careful to do so in limited quantities since it is very easy to overdose on vitamin A.

The main side effect of commercial fish oil supplements is a fishy aftertaste or gastrointestinal disturbances. To overcome this, place the capsules in the refrigerator. Although omega-3 fatty acids have a dose-dependent effect on bleeding time, there are no published cases of abnormal bleeding. There is conflicting evidence for the effect of fish oil on blood sugar control. Most reports state that fish oil does not significantly elevate blood sugar levels.

St. John's Wort

Many MVPers take St. John's wort to help alleviate anxiety, depression, and insomnia, and to help control mood swings. St. John's wort is found in Asia, Europe and the United States. Other names for St. John's wort include goatweed, hardhay, rosin rose, and witches's herb. St. John's wort is reportedly used to treat anxiety, and mild to moderate depression. There are also some reports that St. John's wort is used topically to treat inflammation as in hemorrhoids and burns.

The alcohol extracts of the St. John's wort flower are atypical antidepressants. The active ingredient hypericum is thought to be a weak monoamine oxidase inhibitor (MAOI). The effect of hypericum is to inhibit serotonin reuptake and antagonize reserpine, and inhibit the synaptic gamma-aminobutyric acid (GABA) uptake and GABA-receptor binding. Doses of 117 mg to 250 mg twice a day were shown to be more effective with greater tolerability than imipramine (Tofranil) 75 mg twice a day for the treatment of mild to moderate depression. Side effects are reportedly less with St. John's work as compared to tricyclic antidepressant therapy.

Side effects seen with St. John's wort include rash, constipation, dizziness, restlessness, abdominal cramping, and photosensitivity (sensitivity to light). It is important to know that St. John's wort interacts with a range of medications. In most cases, this interactions leads to reduced effectiveness of the medication; in other cases, however, St. John's wort may increase the effects of a medication. Be certain to inform your health-care provider if you take St. John's wort. Discontinue St. John's wort at least five days before a surgical procedure. Dosage is 300 mg hypericum extract, standardized to 0.3% of hypericin three times a day.

Valerian

Valerian is a perennial that is cultivated throughout the world and is used to treat nervous disorders such as insomnia, anxiety, and restlessness. Its anticonvulsive, sedative, hypotensive and hypnotic effects are believed to occur by binding to the same receptors as benzodiazepines, but with less efficiency and milder effects. Studies report improvement in sleep quality, decreased sleep latency without residual morning sedation. The higher dose (900 mg) seems to have no advantage over the lower dose of 400 mg—the recommended dose.

Side effects of valerian include: restlessness, palpations, headache, and paradoxical stimulation. Overdoses may cause hypothermia, decreased sensibility, ataxia (loss of balance), hallucination, and increased muscle relaxation. On account of these side effects, valerian should not be taken while driving or operating machinery. Drug interactions are not known; however, since valerian is thought to potentate the effect of alcohol, barbiturates, benzodiazepines, and opiates, avoid taking these drugs with valerian. Because of the potential risk of valerian's increasing the sedative effects of anesthesia, valerian should be discontinued before surgery. Caution should be taken with abrupt discontinuation of use in individuals who may be physically dependent on valerian. In these individuals, it may be wise to taper the dose.

Vitamin E

Vitamin E is a fat-soluble vitamin that exists in eight different forms. Each form has its own biological activity, which is the measure of potency or functional use in the body. The most active form of vitamin E in humans is alpha-tocopherol (α-tocopherol), which is also a powerful biological antioxidant. Vitamin E supplements are usually sold as alpha-tocopheryl acetate, a form that protects its ability to function as an antioxidant. The synthetic form is labeled "D, L" while the natural form is labeled "D". The synthetic form is only half as active as the natural form.

Vitamin E is reportedly used for cancer, osteo- and rheumatoid arthritis, and Alzheimer's disease, and to prevent cardiovascular disease. The results of clinical studies have shown promising, albeit mixed, reviews on the efficacy of α-tocopherol in the prevention and treatment of cancer, heart disease and Alzheimer's disease. Although many explanations have been proposed for the lack of consistency in the results of randomized clinical trials, this discussion is beyond the scope of this book.

Dietary vitamin E is obtained mainly from plant sources, including sunflower seeds, olive oil, and almonds. The American Heart Association recommends avoiding doses greater than 400 international units (IU). High doses of vitamin E (greater than 400 IU/day) may increase the risk of bleeding on account of inhibition of platelet aggregation and antagonism of vitamin K–dependent clotting factors. Thus, caution is advised in individuals with bleeding disorders or those who take drugs that may increase the risk of bleeding. Dosing adjustments may be necessary. It is advisable to discontinue vitamin E prior to surgery.

References

Ackermann, R., C. Mulrow, G. Ramirez, C. Gardner, L. Morbidoni & V. Lawrence. 2001. Garlic shows promise for improving some cardiovascular risk factors. *Archives of Internal Medicine* **161**: 813–824.

Amato, P. & D. Marcus. 2003. Review of alternative therapies for treatment of menopausal symptoms. *Climacteric : The Journal of the International Menopause Society* **6**(4): 278–284.

Ang-Lee, M., J. Moss & C. Yuan. 2001. Herbal medicines and perioperative care. *Journal of the American Medical Association* **286:** 2.

Anon. 2004. Echinacea: Cold comfort. *Consumer Reports* **69:** 30–23.

Arad, Y., L. Spadaro, M. Roth, D. Newstein & A. Guerci. 2005. Treatment of asymptomatic adults with elevated coronary calcium scores with atorvastatin, vitamin E: The St. Francis Heart Study randomized clinical trial. *Journal of the American College of Cardiology* **46:** 166–72.

Astin, J. 1998. Why patients use alternative medicine. *Journal of the American Medical Association* **279:** 1548–1553.

Barnes P.M., E. Powell-Griner, K. McFann & R.L. Nahin. Complementary and Alternative Medicine Use among Adults. United States: 2002. Advance Data from Vital and Health Statistics. No 343. Hyattsville, Maryland: National Center for Health Statistics. 2004

Barrett B.P., R.L. Brown, K. Locken *et al.* 2002. Treatment of the common cold with unrefined echinacea: A randomized, double-blind, placebo-controlled trial. *Annals of Internal Medicine* **137**(12): 939–946.

Bloedon, L. & P. Szepary. 2004. Flaxseed and cardiovascular risk. *Nutrition Reviews* **62**: 18–27.

Blumenthal, M., A. Goldberg & J. Brinckmann. 2000. Herbal Medicine: Expanded Commission E Monographs. Integrative Medicine Communication. Newton, MA.

Boerner, R., H. Sommer, W. Berger, U. Kuhn, U. Schmidt & M. Mannel. 2003. Kava-Kava extract LI 150 is as effective as Opipramol and buspirone in generalized anxiety disorder: An 8-week randomized, double-blind multi-centre clinical trial in 129 out-patients. *Phytomedicience* **S IV**: 38–49.

Center for Food Safety and Applied Nutrition, U.S. Food and Drug Administration. Retrieved June 5th, 2005, from http://www.cfsan.fda.gov/~dms/addskava.html.

Clough, A., R. Bailie & B. Currie. 2003. Liver function test abnormalities in users of aqueous Kava extracts. *Journal of Toxicology: Clinical Toxicology* **41**: 821–829.

Covington, M. 2004. Omega-3 fatty acids. *American Family Physician* **70**: 133–140.

Degenring, F., A. Suter, M. Weber & M. Saller. 2003. A randomized double blind placebo controlled clinical trial of a standardized extract of fresh Crateagus berries in the treatment of patients with congestive heart failure NYHA II. *Phytomedincine* **10**: 363–369.

Diaper, A. & I. Hindmarch. 2004. A double blind, placebo-controlled investigation of the effects of two doses of a valerian preparation on the sleep, cognitive and psychomotor function of sleep-disturbed older adults. *Phytotherapy Research* **18**: 831–836.

Eisenberg, D., R. Davis, S. Ettner, S. Appel, S. Wilkey, M. Rompay & R. Kessler. 1998. Trends in alternative medicine use in the United States, 1990–1997: Results of a follow-up national survey. *Journal of the American Medical Association* **280**: 1569–1575.

Gastpar, M. & H. Klimm. 2003. Treatment of anxiety, tension, and restlessness states with Kava special extract WS 1490 in general practice: A randomized placebo-controlled double-blind multicenter trial. *Phytomedicine* **10**: 631–639.

Greeson, J., B. Sanford & D. Monti. 2001. St. John's wort (*Hypericum perforatum*): A review of the current pharmacological, toxicological, and clinical literature. *Psychopharmacology* **153**(4): 402–414.

Foran, J., R. Hites, D. Carpenter, M.C. Hamilton, A. Mathews-Amos & S.J. Schwager. 2004. A survey of metals in tissues of farmed Atlantic and wild Pacific salmon. *Environmental Toxicology and Chemistry/SETAC* **23**(9): 2108–2110.

Fugh-Berman, A. 2003. Echinacea for the prevention and treatment of upper respiratory infections. *Seminars in Integrative Medicine* **1**(2): 106–111.

Harris, W. 2004. Fish oil supplementation: Evidence for health benefits. *Cleveland Clinic Journal of Medicine* **71**: 208–221.

Hofman-Bang, C., N. Rehnqvist, K. Swedberg, I. Wiklund & H. Astrom. 1995. Coenzyme Q10 as an adjunctive in the treatment of chronic congestive heart failure: The Q10 Study Group. *Journal of Cardiac Failure* **2**: 101–107.

Holguin, F., M. Tellez-Rojo, M. Lazo, D. Mannino, J. Schwartz, M. Hernandez & I. Romieu. 2005. Cardiac autonomic changes associated with fish oil versus soy oil supplementation in the elderly. *Chest: The Cardiopulmonary and Critical Care Journal* **127**: 1102–1107.

Hu, F., E. Cho, K. Rexrode, C. Albert & J. Manson. 2003. Fish and long-chain omega fatty acid intake and risk of coronary heart disease and total mortality in diabetic women. *Circulation* **107**: 1852.

Kris-Etherton, P., A. Lichtenstein, B. Howard, D. Steinberg & J. Witztum. 2004. Antioxidant vitamin supplements and cardiovascular disease. *Circulation* **110**: 637–641.

Isaacsohn, J., M. Moser, E. Stein, K. Dudley, J. Davey, E. Liskov & H. Black. 1998. Garlic powder and plasma lipids and lipoproteins: A multicenter, randomized, placebo-controlled trial. *Archives of Internal Medicine* **158**: 1189–1194.

Jenkins, D., C. Kendall, E. Vidgen, S. Agarwal, A. Rao, R. Rosenberg, E. Diamandis, R. Novokmet, C. Mehling, T. Perera, L. Griffin & S. Cunnane. 1999. Health aspects of partially defatted flaxseed, including effects on serum lipids, oxidative measures, and ex vivo androgen and progestin activity: a controlled crossover trial. *American Journal of Clinical Nutrition* **69**: 395–402.

Kiefer, D., S. Shah, P. Gardiner & H. Wechkin. 2001. Finding information on herbal therapy: A guide to useful sources for clinicians. *Alternative Therapy* **7**: 74–78.

Lee, I., N. Cook, M. Gaziano, D. Gordon, P. Ridker, J. Manson, C. Hennekens & J. Buring. 2005. Vitamin E in the primary prevention of cardiovascular disease and cancer: The Women's Health Study: a randomized controlled trial. *Journal of the American Medical Association* **294:** 56–65.

Lemay, A., S. Dodin, N. Kadri, H. Jacques & J. Forest. 2002. Flaxseed dietary supplement versus hormone replacement therapy in hypercholesterolemic menopausal women. *Obstetrics & Gynecology* **100:** 495–504.

Lichtenstein, A. & R. Russell. 2005. Essential nutrients: food or supplements? *Journal of the American Medical Association:* **294:** 3.

Mahady, G., D. Fabricant, L. Chadwick & B. Dietz. 2002. Black cohosh: An alternative therapy for menopause? *Nutrition in Clinical Care* **5:** 283–289.

Masi, M.P. 2003. Bach flower therapy in the treatment of chronic major depressive disorder. *Alternative Therapies in Health and Medicine* **9**(6): 112–110.

Miller, E., R. Pastor-Barriuso, D. Dalal, R. Riemersma, L. Appel & E. Guallar. 2005. Meta-analysis: High-dosage vitamin E supplementation may increase all-cause mortality. *Annals of Internal Medicine* **142:** 37–46.

National Center for Complementary and Alternative Medicine. Retrieved February 1, 2006, from http://nccam.nih.gov/news/camsurvey_fs1.htm.

Office of Dietary Supplements. Retrieved February 1, 2006 from http://ods.od.nih.gov/factsheets/BlackCohosh_pf.asp.

Office of Dietary Supplements. Retrieved February 1, 2006 from http://ods.od.nih.gov/factsheets/vitamine.asp.

PDR for Herbal Medicines. 2000. Medical Economics Company. Montvale, NJ.

Pittler, M., K. Schmidt & R. Ernst. 2003. Hawthorn extract for treating chronic heart failure: Meta-analysis of randomized trials. *American Journal of Medicine* **114:** 665–674.

Polit, D. & C. Beck. 2004. Nursing Research: Principles and Methods. Lippincott Williams & Wilkins. Philadelphia.

Rotblatt, M., and I. Ziment. 2001. Evidence-Based Herbal Medicine. Hanley & Belfus, Inc. Philadelphia.

Rundek, T., A. Naini, R. Sacco, K. Coates & S. DiMauro. 2004. Atorvastatin decreases the coenzyme Q10 level in the blood of patients at risk for cardiovascular disease and stroke. *Archives of Neurology* **61:** 889–892.

Siepmann, M., S. Krause, P. Joraschky, M. Muck-Weymann & W. Kirch. 2002. The effect of St. John's wort extract on heart rate variability, cognitive function and quantitative

EEG: A comparison with amitriptyline and placebo in healthy men. *Journal of Clinical Pharmacology* **54:** 277–282.

Skidmore-Roth, L. 2001. *Mosby's Handbook of Herbs and Natural Supplements.* Mosby, Inc. St. Louis, MO.

Sorensen, H. & J. Sonne. 1996. A double-masked study of the effects of ginseng on cognitive functions. *Current Therapeutic Research* **57:** 959–968.

Sotaniemi, E., E. Haapakoski & A. Rautio. 1995. Ginseng therapy in non-insulin-independent diabetic patients. *Diabetes Care* **18:** 1373–1375.

Spencer, J. & J. Jacobs. 2003. Complementary and Alternative Medication: An Evidence-based Approach. Mosby, Inc. St. Louis, MO.

Taylor J.A., W. Weber, L. Standish, *et al.* 2003. Efficacy and safety of echinacea in treating upper respiratory tract infections in children: A randomized controlled trial. *Journal of the American Medical Association* **290**(21): 2824–2830.

Tesch, B. 2003. Herbs commonly used by women: An evidence-based review. *American Journal of Obstetrics and Gynecology* **188:** S44–S55.

Tessier, D. & D. Bash. 2003. A surgeon's guide to herbal supplements. *Journal of Surgical Research* **114:** 30–36.

The North American Menopause Society. 2004. Treatment of menopause-associated vasomotor symptoms: position statement of The North American Menopause Society. *Menopause* **11**(1): 11–33.

Tucker, J. & M. Townsend. 2005. Alpha-tocopherol: Roles in prevention and therapy of human disease. *Biomedicine & Pharmacotherapy* **59**(7): 380–387.

Veveris, M., U. Koch & S. Chatterjee. 2004. Crataegus special extract WS 1442 improves cardiac function and reduces infarct size in a rat model of prolonged coronary ischemia and reperfusion. *Life Sciences* **74:** 1945–1955.

Walach, H., C. Rilling & U. Engelke. 2001. Efficacy of Bach-flower remedies in test anxiety: A double-blind, placebo-controlled, randomized trial with partial crossover. *Anxiety Disorders* **15:** 359–366.

Weinberg, P. 2005. Analysis of the variable effect of dietary vitamin effect of dietary vitamin E supplement on experimental atherosclerosis. *Journal of Plant Physiology* **162:** 823–833.

Wheatley, D. 2001. Kava and valerian in the treatment of stress-induced insomnia. *Phytotherapy Research* **15:** 549–551.

Wijendran, V. & C. Hayes. 2004. Dietary n-6 and n-3 fatty acid balance and cardiovascular health. *Annual Review of Nutrition* **24:** 597–615.

Yaebe, D. & M. Lievre. 2004. Fish oil in the care of coronary heart disease patients: A meta-analysis of randomized controlled trials. *Fundamental & Clinical Pharmacology* **18:** 581–592.

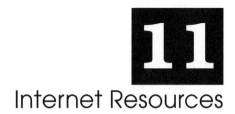

Internet Resources

Many MVPers spend hours surfing the World Wide Web (WWW). They do so to obtain information about MVPS, to converse with other MVPers with similar symptoms, and to find health-care providers sympathetic to their cause. With an endless supply of information, how do you sort fact from fiction? How do you know that the information is accurate and reliable? Think you can trust all that you read? Not so. Anyone can put anything online. Currently there are no standards to guarantee that the content is accurate. So how do you know what you're reading is accurate information? Train your mind to critically think. Ask a series of questions.

This chapter provides a brief description of how to evaluate a health-related website. Many reputable sites are available that give more detailed information on evaluating websites. These are listed at the end of this chapter on page 236. Consumer Internet resources follow this discussion.

Critiquing Websites

Evaluate health-related websites according to the standard criteria: authority, accuracy, objectivity, currency, and coverage. Websites must also be usable and readable; they need to be consistent with Web standards, not printing standards. Find information on usability and readability *Research-Based Web Design & Usability Guidelines* under the Guidelines and Checklist heading at http://www.usability.gov/.

Authority

Currently, any person who wishes to create a health-related website, or any website, may do so. Your task is to distinguish between the reliable and questionable. Whose website is it?

Who are the authors? What are their qualifications? Although there are a number of reputable MVPS websites, be cautious about personal pages; you don't always know the author on many dot-com sites. Individuals claiming to be experts on a particular health-related topic should have readily identifiable academic credentials to support their claims of expertise. You can always "Google" the author. Does the site have a link that allows the consumer to read about the experience of the author as it pertains to the health-related topic? If the website does not provide the name of the author, who is the sponsor of the website—what organization supports the website? Affiliation of a website can often be found in the header or footer. If no affiliation is provided, look at the URL (universal resource locator) address to identify the sponsor and supporting organization. Look for links that say "About us," "Philosophy," "Background," "Biography," "Who am I," etc. If you cannot find these types of links, truncate back the URL. That is, in the top Location Box or URL, delete the end characters of the URL stopping just before each backward slash (leave the slash). Press enter to see if you can see more about the author or the origins/nature of the site providing the page. Continue this process, one slash (/) at a time, until you reach the first single /. This is the page's server or web-site publisher.

Accuracy

Is the information accurate? Are there references? If the content already appeared in peer-reviewed journals such as *Alternative Medicine, Nursing Research, The American Journal of Cardiology, Journal of the American College of Cardiology, Journal of the American Medical Association,* or *The Western Journal of Nursing Research,* it was approved by experts in their field before the article was published.

Identify who sponsored the website and the organization that supports the website. Again, sponsors or organizations of websites are typically identified in the location box or URL address. Remember, a website that contains impressive sound or graphics does not necessarily contain trustworthy information. Here are some common domain names and what they represent.

.com = commercial: URLs that are in this domain represent commercial businesses that are usually trying to sell something, but often contain valuable factual information. It also includes many personal home pages that have .com domains (e.g., geocities.com).

.edu = educational: This does not guarantee that the information will always be authoritative or of research quality. If, on an educational website, you see a "~" followed by a person's name, such as ~lisa.jacobsen, this is a personal web page that is simply located on an educational server. The person is usually a student or employed by the college or university, so their opinions and the contents of their pages may or may not reflect the view of the university they are affiliated with—so be careful when using these pages.

.org = organization: These sites often represent advocacy groups and nonprofit organizations which may have a bias or a particular point of view. Be aware that these sites should always be examined for their particular bias or point of view.

.gov = government: Government agencies often use Internet sites to disseminate statistical and survey information and reports.

.mil = military: These are sites of the United States military.

.net = network organizations: These are directly involved in Internet operations, such as network providers and network information centers. Network sites now often house personal web pages

Country names appear as a two-letter abbreviation in the domain name (e.g., .ie for Ireland, .uk for the United Kingdom). For a complete list, access Domain Name Registries around the World at http://www.norid.no/domenenavnbaser/domreg-alpha.html.

Evaluate the grammar used by the website. Are there misspelled words? The presence of badly spelled, ungrammatical material should raise a red flag.

Accurate websites should be free of grammatical and typographical errors. If spelling, grammar, and punctuation of a site are inaccurate, perhaps the information provided by the website is also inaccurate. What is the purpose of the website? Is it to provide the reader with accurate and reliable health-related information? Accurate health-related websites are not created to entertain the audience but to provide information on a particular health topic.

Objectivity

Is the information objective and free of bias? Does the sponsor or the organization provide factual information? Can consumers make an informed decision based on accurate information, or are they being inflenced in favor of the information provided? Identify advertisements displayed on the website. Websites whose URLs end with dot-com are likely to be biased and often have a primary objective of promoting a particular product, or way of thinking. Websites that use personal testimonials are often attempting to sway the opinion of the reader to their own way of thinking rather than allowing the reader to make a decision based on factual information alone. Remember to ask yourself: Who is providing the testimonials? Do they have any expertise or formal training? Are these paid testimonials? Does the website provide links to organizations or sources where further information may be obtained?

Currency

Is the information up-to-date? Is the page dated? When was the material first written? When was the information first posted? When was it updated? Is the information comparable with that available through other sources? Have the links provided by the website expired or moved? Messages such as "page not found" are not encouraging.

Coverage

What topics are covered and how in-depth is the content? Is the site created for fun or as a hoax? Or does the site provide legitimate information and links to reputable sites that also support the information provided? If the site requires special software to download a file, such as Real Player, PowerPoint, or Adobe Acrobat, are links provided to assist you?

Internet Resources

What follows is a *brief* list of available consumer sites that may be of assistance to you in your search for further knowledge. To obtain a database of thousands of biomedical resources, visit the National Institutes of Health, National Library of Medicine's Health Hotlines at http://dirline.nlm.nih.gov.

Alternative Therapy

American Botanical Council
6200 Manor Rd.
Austin, TX 78723
Tel: (512) 926-4900
Fax: (512) 926-2345
URL: http://www.herbalgram.org

The American Botanical Council (ABC) was established in 1988. It is an independent, nonprofit, international member–based organization that is committed to providing education, both science-based and traditional, in efforts to promote the safe and responsible use of herbal medicine. The ABC serves various audiences including the public, researchers, educators, health-care professionals, industry, and the media.

American Chiropractic Association
1701 Clarendon Boulevard, 2nd Floor
Arlington, VA 22209
URL: http://www.acatoday.com

The ACA is a professional organization that represents Doctors of Chiropractic. Its mission is to preserve, protect, improve and promote the chiropractic profession and the services of Doctors of Chiropractic for the benefit of patients they serve. The purpose of the ACA is to provide leadership in health care and a positive vision for the chiropractic profession and its natural approach to health and wellness. The site has a wealth of information for consumers.

HerbMed
P.O. Box 60016
Potomac, MD 20859
Tel: (301) 340-1960
Fax: (301) 340-1936
http://www.herbmed.org

HerbMed is an interactive, electronic herbal database provided by the nonprofit organization Alternative Medicine Foundation, Inc. This site provides impartial, evidence-based information on the use of herbs to health-care providers, pharmacists, research scientists, health-care consumers, herbal companies, medical writers and advocacy organizations. HerbMed also provides links to numerous medical, scientific, and health websites.

Herb Research Foundation
4140 15th Street
Boulder, CO 80304
Tel: (303) 449-2265
Fax: (303) 449-7849
URL: http://www.herbs.org

The Herb Research Foundation is a non-profit organization that was founded in 1983. The mission of the Herb Research Foundation is to provide research on herbs and public education that promotes truthful information about the health benefits of herbs. The Herb Research Foundation offers a research library that contains more than 300,000 scientific articles on thousands of herbs. Membership packages are available to individuals, professionals, and corporate leaders.

The National Center for Complementary and Alternative Medicine Clearinghouse
P.O. Box 7923,
Gaithersburg, MD 20898-7923
Fax: 1-866-464-3616
Fax-on-Demand service: 1-888-644-6226
Toll-free in the U.S.: 1-888-644-6226
International Tel: 301-519-3153
TTY (for deaf or hard-of-hearing callers): 1-866-464-3615
URL: http://nccam.nih.gov/health/clearinghouse/

The NCCAMC is the public's point of contact for scientifically based information on complementary and alternative medicine (CAM) and for information about NCCAM.

National Center for Homeopathy
PO Box 7923
Gaithersburg, MD 20898-7923
Toll-free in the U.S.: 1-(888) 644-6226
URL: http://www.homeopathic.org

The NCH contains abundant information about homeopathic medicine.

Quackwatch
URL: http://www.quackwatch.com

Quackwatch is a nonprofit corporation whose purpose is to combat health-related frauds, myths, fads, and fallacies. The site offers information about complementary and herbal therapies.

Anxiety and Panic Attacks

American Psychiatric Association
1400 K Street, N.W.
Washington, DC 20005
Tel: (202) 682-6000
URL: http://www.psych.org

A link to consumer resources on this site takes you to Healthy Minds, Healthy Lives, a site that has numerous links related to the recognition and treatment of mental health issues such as anxiety, depression, phobias, and headache.

National Institute of Mental Health
5600 Fishers Lane
Rockville, MD 20857
Tel: (301) 443-4536
URL: http://www.nimh.nih.gov/

The NIMH is a central source of health information for topics that include anxiety disorders and other conditions.

National Mental Health Association
61021 Price Street
Alexandria, VA 22314-2971
Tel: (703) 684-7722
URL: http://www.nmha.org/

The NMHA is the country's oldest and largest nonprofit organization addressing all aspects of mental health and mental illness.

Exercise

American Heart Association
National Center
7272 Greenville Avenue
Dallas, TX 75231
Toll-free: 1-800-AHA-USA-1 or 1-800-242-8721
URL: http://www.americanheart.org/presenter.jhtml?identi-
    fier=1200000

The AHA websites provide information about a variety of health issues, such as heart conditions, nutrition and exercise, for children and adults along with guidelines for exercise.

The American College of Cardiology
Heart House
9111 Old Georgetown Road
Bethesda, MD 20814-1699
Phone: (800) 253-4636, ext. 694, or (301) 897-5400
Fax: (301) 897-9745
URL: http://www.acc.org

This site is mainly geared toward health-care professionals, but guidelines for exercise for many others are provided.

Headaches

American Council for Headache Education
19 Mantua Road
Mount Royal, NH 08061
Tel: (800) 255-2243
URL: http:\\www.achenet.org

The American Council for Headache Education (ACHE) is a non-profit patient–health-care professional partnership dedicated to advancing knowledge about the treatment and management of headache. It also attempts to raise public awareness of headache as a valid, biologically based illness.

National Headache Foundation
820 N. Orleans, Suite 217,
Chicago, IL 60610
Tel: (888) NHF-5552
URL: http://www.headaches.org/

The NHF website provides information for headache sufferers. It also provides links to support groups in your locality and listings of pharmaceuticals to treat headache.

Medications

U.S. Food and Drug Administration
5600 Fishers Lane
Rockville MD 20857-0001
Tel: 1-888-INFO-FDA (1-888-463-6332)
URL: http://www.fda.gov/

The FDA offers a variety of publications on topics such as general drug information and food and nutrition related a variety of subjects.

U.S. Department of Health and Human Services
200 Independence Avenue, S.W.
Washington, D.C. 20201
Tel: 202-619-0257
Toll-free: 1 (877) 696-6775
URL: http://www.hhs.gov/

The DHHS provides information on a variety of health-related topics.

Nutrition

American Dietetic Association
120 South Riverside Plaza, Suite 2000
Chicago, Illinois 60606-6995
Tel: 800/877-1600
URL: http://www.eatright.org

The ADA offers information that is designed to educate the consumer about food and nutrition.

American Diabetic Association
URL: http://www.diabetes.org

This site offers a wealth of valuable information about diabetes as well as understanding the glycemic index. The site is available in Spanish.

Canadian Diabetes Association
URL: http://www.diabetes.ca/

The CDA offers information and answers many questions about diabetes. The site is available in Chinese and French.

The Linus Pauling Institute, Micronutrient Information Center
URL: http://lpi.oregonstate.edu/infocenter/foods/grains/gigl.html

This website is sponsored by Oregon State University and provides links with information on the glycemic index and glycemic load, disease prevention, and various disease states.

Partnership for Essential Nutrition
URL: http://www.essentialnutrition.org/glycemic.php

This website is sponsored by a group of non-profit consumer, nutrition and public health organizations; it offers information about the essentials of a nutritionally balanced diet. Links lead to information on carbohydrates, the glycemic index, and weight loss.

Yale–New Haven Nutrition Advisor
URL: http://www.ynhh.org/online/nutrition/advisor/glycemic_index.html

This site is one of the many links sponsored by Yale–New Haven Hospital. The Nutrition InfoLine offers advice and valuable information about a variety of nutritional topics.

MVPS Support Groups

Friends and Family with Autonomic Nervous System Disorders (FANS) Support Group
Meeting place: St. Luke's Hospital, Maumee, Ohio
Contact: juliatremp@yahoo.com
URL: http://www.potsplace.com/

This website is the Dysautonomia Information Network. Click on support groups to find one in your area.

MVPS Support Group: Austin, Texas
Contact: (512)-692-7631
E-mail: mld@austin.rr.com

New Jersey Self-Help Group Clearinghouse
100 East Hanover Ave., Suite 202
Cedar Knolls, NJ 07927-2020
Tel: (800) 367-6274 or 973-326-6789
URL: http://www.njgroups.org/

The New Jersey Help Group Clearinghouse guides the finding and forming of mutual aid self-help groups.

The Society for Mitral Valve Prolapse Syndrome
P.O. Box 431
Itasca, IL 60143-0431
Tel: (630) 250-9327
URL: http://www.mitralvalveprolapse.com

This site, hosted by individuals with MVPS, provides support and links to resources for MVPers.

Mitral Valve Research and Support Site
E-mail: MVPSupport4@aol.com
URL: http://www.mvpsupport.com/

This site is hosted by an individual with MVPS. It provides support, a message board system, and links to resources for MVPers, where they can research further information.

**Northern Virginia Chronic Fatigue Syndrome and
    Fibromyalgia Support Group**
6507 Columbia Pike
Annadale VA 22003-2029
E-mail: cfsupport-owner@yahoogroups.com
URL: http://www.geocities.com/cfsnova
        http://health.groups.yahoo.com/group/CFSupport/

**Mitral Valve Prolapse Syndrome/Dysautonomia and
    Orthostatic Intolerance Support Group
    of Northern Virginia**
14404 Brookmere Dr.
Centreville, VA 20120-4107
E-mail: MVPS-D_OI_NOVA-owner@yahoogroups.com
URL: http://health.groups.yahoo.com/group/ mvps-d_oi_nova/

The Autonomic Disorders Mitral Valve Prolapse Center
URL: http://www.mvprolapse.com/

The Autonomic Disorders Mitral Valve Prolapse Center provides
general information on understanding MVPS, along with other
resources and a link to support groups.

The Society for Mitral Valve Prolapse Syndrome
Contact: bonnie0107@aol.com
URL: http://www.mitralvalveprolapse.com/INDEX.htm.htm

This site is hosted by individuals with MVPS. Numerous links
provide further information for MVPS.

Women Heart Support Group
Scripps Center for Integrative Medicine
10820 North Torrey Pines Road
La Jolla, CA 92037
Contact: 858-554-3320
URL: http:\\www.scrippsintegrativemedicine.org

Miscellaneous

American Institute for Preventive Medicine
30445 Northwestern Highway, Suite 350
Farmington Hills, MI 48334
Tel: (800) 345-2476
URL: http:\\www.healthylife.com

The AIPM supports the belief that correcting poor health habits is a gradual and systematic process that occurs in a step-wise fashion. The site provides a wealth of information on health promotion programs.

MedlinePlus
U.S. National Library of Medicine
8600 Rockville Pike
Bethesda, MD 20894
Tel: (301) 594-5983
Toll free in the U.S.: (888) 346-3656
URL: http://www.nlm.nih.gov/medlineplus/
    herbalmedicine.html

MedlinePlus is a service of the U.S. National Library of Medicine and the National Institutes of Health. It offers various links pertaining to the safety and use of herbal medicine as well as pictures/diagrams and information about specific conditions, clinical trials, research, and organizations.

Office on Smoking and Health
Centers for Disease Control and Prevention,
1600 Clifton Rd,
Atlanta, GA 30333
Tel: (404) 639-3311
Public inquiries: (404) 639-3534 / (800) 311-3435
URL: http://www.cdc.gov/tobacco/

The OSH serves as a clearinghouse on information about smoking.

National Health Information Clearinghouse
U.S. Department of Health and Human Services
Office of Disease Prevention and Health Promotion
Office of Public Health and Science, Office of the Secretary
1101 Wootton Parkway, Suite LL100
Rockville, MD 20852
Tel: (800)-336-4797
URL: http://www.health.gov/nhic/

The NHIC is a central source of information and referral for
health-related questions of consumers and health professionals. Searches of the database lead to organizational links.

**U.S. National Library of Medicine and the National
     Institutes of Health**
8600 Rockville Pike,
Bethesda, MD 20894
Tel: (888) FIND-NLM
     (888) 346-3656
URL: http://www.nlm.nih.gov/

The NLM is the world's largest biomedical library and educates
users about available sources of information so that they may
conduct their own research concerning medical topics.

Sudden Arrhythmia Death Syndromes Foundation
508 East South Temple, Suite 20
Salt Lake City, UT 84102
Tel: (800) 786-7723
URL: http:\\www.sads.org

This site provides information on arrhythmias and sudden cardiac death.

WWW Resources for Evaluating Internet Resources

**Evaluating Websites: Criteria and Tools—
     Cornell University**

http://www.library.cornell.edu/olinuris/ref/research/
evaluate.html

How To Critically Analyze Information Sources— Cornell University

http://www.library.cornell.edu/okuref/research/skill26.htm

Evaluating Web Resources—Widener University

http://www.widener.edu/Tools_Resources/Libraries/ Wolfgram_Memorial_Library/Evaluate_Web_Pages/659

How Do I Evaluate Information Sources— Wright State University

http://www.libraries.wright.edu/services/tutorials/ termpaper/evaluate4.html

Evaluating Websites—Lesley College:

http://www.lesley.edu/faculty/kholmes/libguides/eval.html

Evaluating Web Pages: Techniques to Apply & Questions to Ask—UC Berkeley

http://www.lib.berkeley.edu/TeachingLib/Guides/Internet/ Evaluate.html

References

Beck, S. 2005. Evaluation criteria. The good, the bad & the ugly: Or why it's a good idea to evaluate web sources. Retrieved January 31, 2006 from http://lib.nmsu.edu/ instruction/evalcrit.html

British Columbia. 2002. BC health files: Evaluating health information on the internet. Retrieved January 31, 2006 from http://www.bchealthguide.org/healthfiles/hfile84.stm

Eysenbach, G., J. Powell, O. Kuss & E. Sa. 2002. Empirical studies assessing the quality of health information for consumers on the World Wide Web: A systematic review. *JAMA* **287**: 2691–2700.

Lang, J.R. & A. Collen. 2005. Evaluating personal health care and health promotion websites. *Methods of Information in Medicine* **44**(2): 328–333.

12

Frequently Asked Questions About MVPS

Since the publication of the first edition of *Taking Control*, we have received countless letters from people all over the world. A compilation of common questions from people who wrote *Network's* column, the Readers' Corner, follows.

How important is it to take antibiotics and why take them?

Although MVPS is a relatively benign condition, one possible complication is infective endocarditis (IE). Infective endocarditis is a bacterial infection of the heart valve(s) or lining of the heart. It occurs when bacteremia—bacteria in the bloodstream—lodge on an abnormal heart valve or other damaged tissue. In MVP, mechanical stress and turbulent blood flow may injure a valve's surface and create an opportunity for bacteria in the blood stream to deposit on the valve. The bacteria cause wart-like growths that can damage and even destroy the heart valve.

Certain heart conditions place a person at a greater risk for developing endocarditis when a bacteremia occurs. Some of these conditions include:

- prostheses—artificial heart valves
- certain congenital cardiac malformations
- valvular heart disease—such as valves damaged by rheumatic fever and other acquired valve dysfunction
- mitral valve prolapse with documented valvular regurgitation—back flow of blood through the opening of the mitral valve leaflets—and/or valvular thickening
- hypertrophic cardiomyopathy—heart muscle disease
- a history of previous bacterial endocarditis, even in the absence of heart disease

Bacteria commonly enter the bloodstream during certain surgical procedures that involve contaminated tissue, and during dental procedures that may cause gingival (gum) bleeding. This causes a transient, brief bacteremia that rarely lasts for more than 15 minutes. Only a limited number of types of bacteria commonly cause endocarditis. It is impossible to predict, however, which person will develop an infection—or which particular procedure will be responsible. Unless there are antibiotics in the blood to combat the bacteria, this bacteremia can cause endocarditis.

Since the 1950's, the American Heart Association (AHA) has published guidelines for the prevention of bacterial endocarditis. The latest guidelines were published in *JAMA* on June 11, 1997. In general, antibiotic prophylaxis is recommended for all

---

PROCEDURES FOR WHICH ENDOCARDITIS PROPHYLAXIS IS INDICATED INCLUDE*

- Dental procedures known to induce gum bleeding including professional cleaning (but not simple adjustment of orthodontic appliances or natural loss of a tooth)

- Tonsillectomy and/or adenoidectomy

- Surgical procedures or biopsy involving respiratory mucosa

- Bronchoscopy with a rigid bronchoscope

- Sclerotherapy of esophageal varices

- Esophageal dilatation

- Gallbladder surgery

- Cystoscopy

- Urethral dilatation

- Urethral catheterization if urinary tract infection is present

- Prostatic surgery

- Incision and drainage of infected tissue

- Vaginal hysterectomy

- Vaginal delivery in the presence of infection

---

*From Dajani *et al.* 1997

HELPFUL TIPS WHEN TAKING ANTIBIOTICS

- Obtain the handy wallet-size card from your local chapter of the American Heart Association or physician's office. The card lists the antibiotics and dosage commonly prescribed. Ask your physician to circle the one he recommends, and also list your diagnosis in the space provided. Complete the top of the card with your name, address, and telephone number. Carry this card with you.

- Before any procedure, ask about the need for taking antibiotics. Not every procedure requires them.

- Take the antibiotic on an empty stomach to increase the absorption in the small intestine.

- If you experience stomach upset, nausea, or vomiting when taking amoxicillin, take it with a little food or milk to "buffer" it. Be sure to check with the dentist to see if you are allowed a small amount of food.

- If your stomach is upset from erythromycin, get the enteric coated form. It's kinder to your stomach.

- Antacids decrease drug absorption. Do not take them with antibiotics.

- Alert your physician, pharmacist, nurse practioner, physician's assistant to all medications you take—especially if you plan to be on antibiotics for any length of time. Many drugs interact with antibiotics.

- To avoid diarrhea, take *Lactobacillus* tablets—available in many health food stores—or eat four to eight ounces of yogurt daily. Be certain the yogurt contains *live yogurt cultures*. Some refrigerated brands contain live cultures. Frozen yogurt does not.

- Maintain good oral hygiene, and see your dentist regularly. When bleeding occurs with tooth brushing, bacteria that enter the blood stream are usually not sufficient to cause endocarditis. It is, however, important to not let the bacteria build up in your mouth. Brush and floss on a regular basis.

- Report symptoms such as: malaise, fatigue, loss of appetite, fever, or weight loss. These are common symptoms of endocarditis, and they usually start within two weeks of the precipitating bacteremia.

dental procedures likely to cause gingival bleeding, even for routine, routine professional cleaning. Antibiotics are also recommended for surgery, instrumentation, or diagnostic procedures that involve the genitourinary or gastrointestinal tracts, such as gallbladder surgery, bronchoscopy, and incision and drainage of infected tissue.

The recommended standard drug for all *dental, oral,* and *upper respiratory tract procedures* is amoxicillin. To be effective, 2 grams of amoxicillin should be taken by mouth one hour before the procedure. For people who are allergic to penicillins (such as amoxicillin, ampicillin, or penicillin) clindamycin or azithromycin is used. The dose is 600 mgm of clindamycin one hour before the procedure, or 500 mgm azithromycin one hour before the procedure. Antibiotic prophylaxis is also recommended for children with MVP. The dose of antibiotic is based on the weight of the child.

How do you know whether you need antibiotics?

First and foremost—always verify this with your health-care provider.

Usually this is discussed when you are first diagnosed. The AHA recommends antibiotics for people with MVP and valvular regurgitation or insufficiency—a backflow of blood and/or thickened leaflets. This backflow of blood causes a murmur—an extra heart sound. Regurgitation is visible on a color flow (2D) echocardiographic examination. Therefore, people with MVP who have a murmur should take antibiotics prophylactically. Other health-care professionals recommend antibiotics if you have a click, or extra heart sounds. Recommendations for antibiotic prophylaxis for MVP continue to be controversial; the recommendations are still evolving.

Again, always consult your health-care professional to verify the need for antibiotics.

Can people with MVP safely use water-picks to clean their teeth? Would some gum bleeding be safe during the use of this device?

Water-picks are small hose-like devices that produce a stream of water to irrigate the teeth and supporting structures.

Although a water-pick *does not* take the place of brushing and flossing, it cleans well around fixed bridges and helps maintain good oral hygiene.

To answer the question: Yes, people with MVP may brush, floss, and use a water-pick *if they have good oral health.*

On the other hand, people with MVP who have periodontal disease—indicated by gum bleeding—must exercise caution. They can inadvertently introduce bacteria into the blood stream by brushing, flossing and using a water-pick. It is extremely important, therefore, that MVPers work closely with their dentist.

What effect does MVPS have on pregnancy?

According to available data and clinical experience, women with MVPS need not anticipate complications during pregnancy. In fact, the frequency of complications is no greater in women with MVP than those without MVP.

Women frequently report an increase in their symptoms during the early part of pregnancy. At approximately two months' gestation, however, circulatory blood volume rapidly increases. This expansion of intravascular volume causes symptoms related to a low circulating blood volume—a forceful heart beat and/or dizziness upon standing—to become less evident. Also, the click and murmur—physical findings associated with MVP—sometimes disappear.

Physicians' recommendations for antibiotic prophylaxis—preventive treatment—sometimes vary. Although available data suggests antibiotic prophylaxis may not be necessary for an uncomplicated vaginal delivery, many obstetricians prefer to give antibiotics to all women who had a murmur prior to pregnancy.

Because of highly mobile joints associated with MVP, it has been suggested that delivery might be easier. However, no evidence supports this hypothesis.

What is the natural history of MVP?

MVP has a relatively benign course and excellent prognosis for most people, with a survival rate similar to that in an age-matched and sex-matched population without MVP. A minority of persons, however, develop serious complications. These include infective endocarditis, cerebrovascular events, progressive severe mitral regurgitation, arrhythmias and sudden cardiac death. The risk of complications is highest in men, individuals older than 45 years, persons with familial MVP, and those with left-sided chamber enlargement.

How great is my risk of sudden death?

Clinical studies identify two distinct groups of people with mitral valve prolapse. First, is the younger group (individuals in their 30's and 40's) predominantly female, and with symptoms unrelated to valvular dysfunction—the mitral valve prolapse syndrome. Second, is the older group (individuals over 50, predominantly male) with symptoms of valvular dysfunction who frequently require mitral valve surgery—anatomic MVP. The incidence of sudden death is believed to differ between these two groups.

Mitral Valve Prolapse Syndrome

Thus far, research suggests that sudden death in people with mitral valve prolapse who do not have significant mitral regurgitation—back flow of blood into the left atrium or top chamber—is uncommon. Fewer than a hundred cases have been reported in the literature. Since 4–5% of the population—or close to seven million people—have mitral valve prolapse, the incidence of sudden death is very low.

For comparison, the annual risk of sudden death among the *entire* adult U.S. population is estimated at 300,000 per year, mostly due to coronary artery disease. This translates into an overall incidence of sudden death of 10 to 20/10,000 population, or 0.1–0.2% per year. Compare this to the risk of sudden death for MVPS at 2/10,000 population per year, or .02%. The low risk for sudden death among people with MVPS without significant mitral regurgitation is compatible with the belief that uncomplicated MVPS is inherently a benign—neutral—finding.

Anatomic Mitral Valve Prolapse

The development of significant mitral regurgitation, a complication of *anatomic* MVP, occurs in 2 to 4% of people with mitral valve prolapse. This complication occurs more commonly in men above 50 years of age. The risk of sudden death in this group, although controversial, is *estimated* at 94 to 188 per 10,000, or 1–2% a year, quite different from those without significant mitral regurgitation. This older group has a higher prevalence of complex ventricular arrhythmias—or disturbances in the heart's rhythm—along with depressed pumping action of the heart muscle. These complex arrhythmias and depressed heart function, together with significant mitral regurgitation, are believed to place this group of people with MVP at a higher risk for sudden death.

Thus, current studies suggest that, although sudden death does occur, it is uncommon among those with MVPS. Although certain predictors of sudden death are not clearly identified, people who *may* be at a higher risk include those with a history of recurrent syncope (passing out), a history of sustained supraventricular arrhythmias, complex ventricular arrhythmias (repetitive short runs of extra beats), or a family history of cardiac sudden death. Thus far, no single finding or combination of findings proves to be a consistent predictor of sudden death.

Will the valve have to be replaced?

This is a common question. Natural history studies indicate that people with MVPS with symptoms unrelated to the valve have a relatively benign prognosis—a normal life span. They rarely require valve replacement. Valve surgery is usually reserved for those with severe mitral regurgitation and/or decreased pumping action of the heart (reduced left ventricular function) regardless of symptoms.

Will the extra heart sound or sounds always be heard on physical examination?

It is well known that MVP is a very dynamic syndrome. The findings on cardiac auscultation—listening to heart sounds—sometimes vary from one examination to another. Due to changes in blood volume within the heart, either or both the click and murmur, diagnostic of MVP, sometimes may not be heard. Likewise, if you are well hydrated, and on beta-blockers or tranquilizers, neither a click nor a murmur may be audible.

Will the echocardiogram *always* show the MVP?

An echocardiogram (ultrasound) is used to confirm the diagnosis of MVP. The mitral valve, however, may not be optimally visualized. Sometimes it is difficult to obtain a clear picture of the valve. At other times, MVP may be present, but not seen on the echocardiogram. This is known as a false-negative result.

Usually, if MVP is seen on the echocardiogram, it will be seen on future tests. Negative findings at a later date may be due to either or both inadequate visualization of the mitral valve or the use of different diagnostic criteria by the physician reader. Although manifestations of MVP vary from day to day, the use of strict echocardiographic criteria can avoid misdiagnosis and help to remove the uncertainty of knowing whether or not MVP is present.

Do the more symptoms I have mean the worse the valve is?

No. In MVPS, there is no correlation between the amount of symptoms an individual has and the degree to which the valve buckles back.

Is it safe to take birth control pills if I have MVPS?

Birth control pills (BCPs) sometimes alter the blood-clotting system and increase the risk of cerebrovascular accidents, such as a stroke. This risk may be increased by concomitant cigarette use, high blood pressure, and the use of birth control pills with high estrogen content.

Although the issue of MVP and BCPs is not clearly defined, anyone who has suffered any of the following embolic events would be wise to avoid BCPs: cerebral embolism (blood clot to the brain), pulmonary embolism (blood clot to the lungs), or transient ischemic attack (TIA).

What may place an individual with MVP at a higher-than-normal risk for cerebral embolism? A combination of cigarette smoking, severe migraine headaches, thickened mitral valve leaflets—seen on the echocardiogram—and birth control pills. *It is recommended that you discuss this with your physician.*

Is it safe to donate blood if I have MVPS?

For most individuals with MVPS, donating blood is not contraindicated: it is not dangerous or undesirable. On the other hand, those who have severe orthostatic hypotension—lowering of the blood pressure upon standing—or those sensitive to volume depletion, should not give blood.

Before giving blood, however, check with your physician first. If you do donate blood, drink plenty of fluids prior to and after the procedure.

What about getting life insurance? Should I check heart disease?

Unfortunately, not everyone is well versed on MVPS. John Q. Public sees the word "valve" and often associates it with a heart disease that carries a different prognosis. Then, some people find it difficult to obtain insurance. Others sometimes even pay higher rates as high-risk individuals.

You are frequently asked, "Do you have heart disease?" Yes, MVP, a valvular disease, falls under the general heading of heart disease. Likewise, *heart disease* and *coronary artery disease*, although they differ in meaning, come under the same general heading.

Do you have a heart murmur? Do not assume because of MVP you have a murmur. Many MVPers have a click without a murmur so ask your physician. Computerized cross referencing between insurance companies and physicians' offices has become sophisticated. Honesty is the best policy.

Next, as you shop around for an insurance policy, carefully read any policy that appeals to you. Contact your insurance agent or the insurance company for answers to questions. In spite of frustrations, continue your search. As an informed consumer who diligently shopped, you'll eventually find the policy that fits your budget and your needs. Also, if necessary, ask your physician to discuss in a short letter MVP and its prognosis. It may help.

Should I have my children checked for MVP?

Often, MVP in children is diagnosed as the result of a routine physical examination. The physician hears a click or murmur. However, silent MVP—normal heart sounds—does occur. An echocardiogram confirms the diagnosis. Follow-up includes yearly physical examinations, echocardiograms, and antibiotic prophylaxis.

To a lesser extent, children and adolescents have symptoms similar to those in adults. Chest pain, palpitations, and shortness of breath are common. The cause of the symptoms remains unknown.

Remember, children are impressionable. Therefore, assure them their condition is not uncommon, and that it is treatable. Also, children learn by example. Have you seen children playing, pretending to be parents? The experience is enlightening. If the parent stays in bed all day and conveys a feeling of fear, expect children to do so. Strive to be a good role model with healthy attitudes and behavior patterns.

How can I be sure that the chest pain is not from coronary artery disease?

The answer to this relates to your original diagnosis. To first determine whether heart disease is present, your physician considers your cardiovascular risk factors, symptoms, and diagnostic testing results. Periodically, follow up with testing such as an exercise stress test in order to reassure yourself that the chest pain is not caused by coronary artery disease.

I seem to be more flexible than other people. Is this part of MVPS?

As a child, could you assume a yoga position more easily than your friends could? Could you bend your fingers way back and also perform other contortions? Increased joint flexibility, commonly associated with MVP, theoretically relates to a generalized alteration of connective tissue. Connective tissue is found in tendons, ligaments, and muscles. One of its major components is collagen. Collagen—a protein—is a tough, fibrous material that provides strength to various structures within the body. There are a number of different types of collagen. Changes in the composition of these collagen types, found in connective tissue, enhance joint flexibility.

Why are MVPS symptoms more frequent and intense when I am sick with a cold, flu, or an infection?

Various stressors, whether with a physiological basis such as infection, or with a psychological basis such as emotional stress, can worsen MVPS symptoms. For example, during menses, many women report their symptoms either intensify or surface more frequently. Stressors, such as arthritic pain or infections, affect a number of bodily systems, one of which is the autonomic nervous system. Over-sensitivity of this system is believed to cause a number of the symptoms associated with MVPS.

When you are ill, it is important to continue non-drug symptom control. In other words, maintain an adequate fluid intake. Avoid caffeinated products and medications that contain adrenaline-like substances. Get adequate rest. Do not overexert yourself. Overexertion—particularly when you are ill—prolongs recovery. Once you feel better, begin exercising to a perceived exertion of *fairly light*. Shortly afterward, gradually increase the intensity of your workload to a perceived exertion of *somewhat hard*. The better conditioned you are, the easier it becomes to bounce back.

What medications may I safely use when I have a cold, or when my allergies worsen?

Not all MVPers react the same. Many experience increased symptoms when they use antihistamines or decongestants. Therefore, never randomly select an over-the-counter medication. But, don't despair. There are prescription medications that offer relief of cold or allergy symptoms without increasing MVPS symptoms.

Antihistamines

Antihistamines are medications that interfere with histamine, a culprit responsible for sneezing, a stuffy nose, a runny nose, and itching eyes, all of which are associated with allergies. Antihistamines prevent rather than reverse the actions of histamines. For maximum effectiveness, take medication one to two hours *before* anticipated exposure to the offending allergen. Example: If you're allergic to cut grass, take an antihistamine at least one hour before you walk in a recently mowed area.

The anticholinergic properties of these drugs cause the drying effects of antihistamines. An anticholinergic blocks or interferes with the action of the parasympathetic nervous system—the decelerator. For some MVPers, these anticholinergic effects also cause tachycardia—fast heart beat and palpitations. Also, because antihistamines may have a sedative effect, they can cause drowsiness.

Not all antihistamines are alike. Different agents have varying sedative and anticholinergic effects. Antihistamines with little or no central or autonomic nervous system effects are now available. These drugs have either minimal or no sedative or anticholinergic effects. They include fexofenadine (Allegra™) and desloratadine (Clarinex™) and cetirizine (Zyrtec™). MVPers who noted increased symptoms with over-the-counter antihistamines seem to do better with these medications.

Decongestants

Decongestants are sympathomimetic agents. They mimic the action of the sympathetic nervous system—the accelerator. Therefore, they can cause palpitations, a rapid heart beat, and nervous feeling. Unlike antihistamines, these drugs are mostly used to relieve symptoms related to colds and allergies. Studies associated with people not known to have MVPS report that decongestants with pseudoephedrine hydrochloride are reasonable safe at dosages less than 180 mg. According to studies, in higher doses, however, pseudoephedrine raised blood pressure and heart rate in normal subjects. Although no studies have been conducted in people with MVPS, if you must take a decongestant choose one with the lowest dose of pseudoephedrine hydrochloride.

Is there a relationship between symptoms and work schedules?

Yes, it's not unusual for symptoms to worsen if you job is very stressful. For example, does it require rotating shifts and long hours? Are you unhappy with your position? If so, learn to help yourself in other ways, such as stress management and non-drug symptom control interventions.

Do other people with MVPS complain of increased symptoms due to insufficient sleep?

Yes. It is not unusual for people with MVPS to complain of sleeplessness caused by insomnia, anxiety, or palpitations. Lack of sleep causes even more fatigue, irritability, and a host of other complaints. Any type of stress—including sleeplessness—can potentially increase symptoms associated with MVPS.

To hasten sleep, avoid eating highly acidic foods, such as tomatoes and citrus fruits, late at night. Also, avoid alcohol—particularly wine. While it quickly brings on sleep, it awakens you in the middle of the night. Furthermore, alcohol, along with insufficient water intake can also lead to dehydration, fatigue, headaches, and disturbed sleep.

Known stimulants such as: caffeine, nicotine, and foods high in sugar also cause sleeplessness. Wind down a few hours before you retire. Relax, watch TV, listen to the radio, or read. Learn *how* to effectively deal with everyday stressors. Also, get regular cardiovascular exercise. Those MVPers who exercise on a regular basis enjoy better sleep patterns.

Does a person's weight have anything to do with having symptoms of MVP?

Thus far, no published studies address a relationship between a person's weight and the degree of MVP symptoms. People of all shapes and sizes suffer from symptoms to varying degrees. From clinical observations, however, thinner people with MVPS frequently have lower blood pressures. Their pressure may further decrease whenever they rise, from either a lying or a sitting position. Then, along with a compensatory increase in heart rate, they feel lightheaded, and they note a forceful heartbeat. This reaction may be partly related to a decreased intravascular volume—the volume of blood contained within the circulatory system.

Theoretically, obesity can worsen MVPS symptoms. Frequently, obese individuals are in poor cardiovascular condition. This leads to higher resting heart rates and inappropriate increases in heart rate with minimal activities. Both contribute to fatigue.

I know I am supposed to exercise, but how can I when I'm exhausted?

Listen to an MVP program participant. "I believe the exercise program greatly decreased my MVP symptoms. During the first four weeks of exercise, my symptoms remained constant. I experienced heart palpitations, dizziness, and fatigue daily. I became frustrated, unmotivated, and anxious. I wanted immediate results.

"During the fifth and sixth weeks, I experienced heart palpitations only three or four days each week—not daily.

"As the weeks passed, I became less dizzy as I arose from a seated position. Also, after twelve weeks, I feel less tired by night, and no longer take a lengthy, daily rest. Too, I am less moody and less irritable.

"In every way, this exercise program offers a positive experience. I am in much better physical condition and in greater control of my MVP symptoms. I highly recommend exercise—it is invaluable."

Remember, Rome was not built in a day. Don't expect miracles overnight. Give it time, and you WILL start to feel better.

I recently moved. How can I find a physician?

MVPers recommend the following ideas:

- Ask friends to help. Someone knows someone else who knows a physician to recommend.

- Call a local hospital and ask to speak to a nurse in the coronary care unit or the cardiac step-down unit. Explain that you are new to the area and in need of a cardiologist. Ask if she would please recommend someone. These units tend to be very busy. *Please understand this if someone cannot assist you at that moment; ask if you may leave your phone number, or else call again.*

- Contact your local cardiac rehabilitation facility.

- Call the local Academy of Medicine

- Call a local women's club

- Speak to people at the YWCA or YMCA

- Check the local paper for a class or symposium on a heart-health related topic where the speaker is a physician

- Call your local "Ask a Nurse" program or a physician-referral source. These services are usually organized by local hospitals.

- Call your local Welcome Wagon organization

- Call the local women's center, such as Women Helping Women, or one at an area hospital

- Call a local MVP support group member

When I have a skipped beat, it feels like my heart stopped. Does it?

No, it doesn't stop.

Skipped or extra beats are very common among MVPers *and* the general public. Premature ventricular contractions (PVCs) frequently cause this sensation. While some people feel each beat, others are unaware of them. PVCs sometimes occur following the use of caffeine, alcohol, or certain medications. Emotional stress and smoking may also cause PVCs.

Premature ventricular contractions are beats that come ahead of the normal electrical sequence. When a premature beat occurs, the heart doesn't fill with its normal amount of blood. Thus, the contraction is less forceful than normal. To compensate for this early beat, the heart pauses. This pause—a compensatory pause—gives the heart a longer time to fill. What you feel, therefore, is the normal compensatory pause.

When should a person, as a last alternative, consider medication for heart palpitations?

The answer to this question depends upon the type of rhythm problem that causes palpitations and your symptoms. With MVP, one treats the symptoms, not the valve. Therefore, unlike antibiotics that cure infections, medications do not cure MVP. Many MVPers reported they continue to have symptoms even with medications. Others said they felt worse after starting medication. No studies support the positive effects of medication on MVP symptoms.

Not all MVPers require medication. Occasional extra beats, or flip-flops, although annoying and frightening, seldom require medication. Consuming adequate amounts of salt and water often alleviates the pounding sensation—or forceful heartbeat—noted upon standing. People with rhythm disturbances, however, such as atrial fibrillation, or episodes of passing out due to arrhythmias—disturbance in the heart's rhythm—usually require medication. *Discuss the need for medication with your physician.*

What causes this feeling of fogginess I have?

Several MVPers complain about this feeling. Some say they have a hard time remembering what they are supposed to remember, and feel as if they are in a daze. No one knows the reason. Some MVPers believe lack of sleep worsens their fogginess.

Can smoking make MVP symptoms worse?

Nicotine stimulates the sympathetic nervous system and affects the cardiovascular system. Theoretically, smoking can aggravate symptoms associated with MVPS. Also, cigarette smoking transiently increases the adhesiveness of platelets, accelerates the heart rate, and raises the blood pressure. At the same time, the oxygen carrying capacity of the blood is reduced. Smoking is the leading cause of cardiovascular morbidity and mortality in the United States. It accounts for 30 to 40% of deaths from coronary artery disease. Smoking increases the incident of a heart attack and related death by 70%. For women taking oral contraceptives, cigarette smoking markedly predisposes to cardiovascular disease.

Smoking is one of the highest risk factors for cardiovascular disease, yet the most preventable. It is a bad idea, especially for those with MVP.

Can I live without taking my anti-anxiety medication such as alprazolam (Xanax)?

Yes, of course you can.

No one has to take Xanax or other anti-anxiety medication. People who experience anxiety and panic attacks need to consciously and clearly establish priorities. If the highest priority in your life is not to take medication—especially none that is potentially addicting—then, aim to win the war against that insidious enemy ... Xanax. Use it only when you absolutely *have to*. Otherwise, you may feel defeated when you *do* use it, and become even more anxious about needing it again. This thought process increases your baseline anxiety level, and in turn, increases the frequency of your panic attacks. To focus solely on the medication, you avoid the real causes of your anxiety and the games continue.

When you establish *yourself* as your top priority, and make *your* quality of life a goal, then Xanax, or other anti-anxiety medication, is useful as an occasional aid. With your nervous system stabilized, and panic attack symptoms controlled, you're better equipped—physically and emotionally—to consider the core issues that set your nervous system off like a brass band.

There are reasons for your panic attacks that you must address. First, however, the frightening and immobilizing symptoms have to be treated. Xanax, or similar medication, is effective *short-term* treatment for the symptoms. To rely on medication and to not address the cause of your symptoms is a disservice to you and to the medication. Decide that YOU deserve something better in life.

References

Boudoulas, H., P. Kligfield & C. Wooley. 1988. Mitral valve prolapse: Sudden death. *In* Mitral Valve Prolapse and the Mitral Valve Prolapse Syndrome. H. Boudoulas & C. Wooley, Eds.: 591–605. Futura Publishing Co. Mount Kisco, NY.

Dajani, A., A. Bisno, K. Chung, *et al.* 1990. Prevention of bacterial endocarditis: Recommendations by the American Heart Association. *Journal of the American Medical Association* **262**(22): 2919–2922.

Devereux, R., R. Kramer-Fox, K. Shear & P. Kligfield. 1994. The relation of panic attacks and midsystolic murmurs to the diagnosis of mitral valve prolapse. *Cardiovascular Reviews & Reports*, April 11–15, p. 34.

Eckman, J. 1991. Reader's corner. *Network* **3**(1): 2.

Hayek, E. & B. Griffin. 2002. Mitral valve prolapse: Old beliefs yield to new knowledge. *Cleveland Journal of Medicine* **69:** 889–896.

Hussey, L. 1992. What about Xanax? Part I. *Network* **4**(2): 1.

Kligfield, P., D. Levy, R. Devereux, *et al.* 1987. Arrhythmias and sudden death in mitral valve prolapse. *American Heart Journal* **113:** 1298–1307.

Kligfield, P. & R. Devereux. 1990. Is the mitral valve prolapse patient at high risk of sudden death identifiable? *Cardiovascular Clinics* **21**(1): 143–157.

Kolibash, A. 1988. Natural history of mitral valve prolapse. *In* Mitral Valve Prolapse and the Mitral Valve Prolapse Syndrome. H. Boudoulas & C. Wooley, Eds.: 257–288. Futura Publishing Co. Mount Kisco, NY.

Lax, D., M. Eicher, M. & S. Goldberg. 1993. Effects of hydration on mitral valve prolapse. *American Heart Journal* **126**(2): 415–418.

Myerburg, R. & A. Castellanos. 1992. Cardiac arrest and sudden cardiac death. *In* Heart Disease: A Textbook of Cardiovascular Medicine, 4th ed. E. Braunwald, Ed.: 756–789. W.B. Saunders Co. Philadelphia.

Ohara, N., T. Mikajima, J. Takagi & H. Kato. 1991. Mitral valve prolapse in childhood: The incidence and clinical presentations in different age groups. *Acta Paediat. Jpn.* **33:** 467–475.

Reginelli, J. & B. Griffin. 2004. The challenge of valvular heart disease: When is it time to operate? *Cleveland Journal of Medicine* **6:** 463–486.

Savage, D., Garrison, R., Devereux, R. et al. (1983). Mitral valve prolapse in the general population. I. Epidemiologic features: The Framingham Study. *American Heart Journal* **106:** 571.

Utz, S. & B. England. 1993. Avoiding problems when taking antibiotics. *Network* **5**(3): 1.

13
Summary

MVPS—mitral valve prolapse syndrome—is a common clinical condition that affects millions of people. Anatomic MVP—mitral valve prolapse—occurs when one or more mitral valve leaflets buckle back or prolapse into the left atrium as the heart contracts. Anatomic MVP is often associated with a constellation of symptoms, such as fatigue, dizziness, palpitations, headaches, lightheadedness, chest pain, and panic attacks. Individuals with one or more of these symptoms are referred to as having mitral valve prolapse *syndrome.*

The term MVP syndrome refers to the occurrence or coexistence of symptoms unexplainable on the basis of the valvular abnormality. *Thus, symptoms associated with MVPS are not due to the valve itself.* They are believed to be based on various physiological changes.

Often these symptoms are frightening, discomforting, frustrating, and incapacitating. They can alter one's lifestyle, result in absenteeism from work, and cause disharmony within the family. Visits to an emergency room or a physician's office become quite common and nerve-racking.

Further research is needed to define methods of long-term treatment of MVPS. There are, however, non-drug interventions that effectively decrease the frequency and the severity of symptoms. Developed from information extrapolated from previous research studies, and from years of clinical experience, some recommendations include regular cardiovascular exercise, an increase in sodium and fluid intake, and an avoidance of caffeine and over-the-counter medications that contain adrenaline-like substances.

In conclusion, this book provides you with information to better understand MVPS: what it is, what causes symptoms, and *what you can do to help yourself.* With knowledge comes power—the power to take control of your life.

NOW, DO IT!

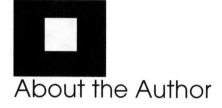

About the Author

Kristine A. Bludau Scordo received her Ph.D. and Master's degrees from The Ohio State University, undergraduate degrees from the University of Cincinnati and Mercy College, New York, and her RN diploma from Queens General Hospital, New York City. She is professor and director of the Acute Care Nurse Practitioner Program, Wright State University, Dayton, OH, former Clinical Director of the Mitral Valve Prolapse Program of Cincinnati, and is a cardiac acute care nurse practitioner at Schuster Cardiology & Associates, Dayton, Ohio. Dr. Scordo is a widely published researcher, author, editor, and lecturer.

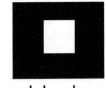

Subject Index